The Big Cookbook with Real Food for Pregnancy

The Guidebook for Pregnancy with 150 Delicious Recipes for an Optimal Prenatal Nutrition

Christine Rosenstein

1st edition

2021

Table of Contents

Appetizers 113

Introduction

When you hold this book in your hands, you are most likely one of the women who are currently experiencing the miracle of pregnancy. Congratulations! There is probably hardly any event in a woman's life that is as formative and amazing as the growing life in her own womb.

Your body changes, the hormones go crazy in the most positive sense and somehow you are surprised how your body changes all of a sudden and how it suddenly behaves. What an exciting time! Morning nausea, exhaustion and constant tiredness are only some of the accompanying symptoms that can accompany you for several weeks or months, especially at the beginning.

If this is your first pregnancy, you are certainly excited and wondering what you can do to make it as easy as possible for you and your baby to get pregnant and give your child the best possible start in life. Perhaps a little fear and uncertainty is mixed in with the feeling of doing something wrong. Don't worry - this is all normal and is also a part of the process of becoming a mother.

I am delighted to be able to support you in this very special phase of your life and to accompany you in the form of this guide. The information you will receive in this book will certainly answer many of your questions and give you more confidence about how to behave best.

On the following pages, you can learn about the great influence your diet and behavior have on the healthy development of your baby. Some of this information will be familiar to you, but you will certainly also learn interesting facts that you did not know before. Immerse yourself in the world of vitamins and nutrients, fats and minerals and find out which of them your body needs so urgently right now.

Are you afraid that you could be plagued by ravenous appetite attacks, heartburn and back pain? Here you will find helpful tips on what you can do about it yourself. Explained in detail and in a way that is easy to understand, you will not only find the optimal diet for the three trimesters in this guide, but also find out which problems can (but do not have to) occur during pregnancy and how you can often help yourself with small measures.

Be curious about which foods you should definitely eat at this special phase of your life and which foods you should avoid at all costs in order to protect your and your child's health and promote their development in the best possible way.

We will once and for all dispel the myth that during pregnancy you have to eat "for 2" and in the process we will also look at the issue of "weight gain". Because this inevitably goes along with pregnancy. You would like to integrate all this theoretical knowledge into your everyday life but don't really know how? Nothing easier than that! In addition to all this valuable information, you will also find numerous tasty and simple recipes that you can easily prepare yourself during your pregnancy. This is quasi "learning by doing" in its pure form!

You can look forward to this and much more on the following pages. Enjoy the exciting time ahead of you and prepare yourself for the growing life in your belly with optimal nutrition during pregnancy.

We hope you enjoy reading, learning and trying out.

Why healthy nutrition is so important

Basically, we all know it and it is almost on everyone's lips: A healthy diet is essential if you want to become or remain healthy, fit and vital. It should be rich in nutrients, contain little sugar and fat, but plenty of vitamins, proteins and fiber. All this is already well known and I am not saying anything new.

If one is as woman however now in this exciting phase of a pregnancy, the topic nutrition gets however again completely different meaning. Now the woman is no longer only responsible for her own health, but also for that of the unborn life in her womb. This is indeed quite a challenge.

Everything that the mother-to-be ingests in liquid and solid food is inevitably transferred to the unborn child through the umbilical cord. In the best case, the baby now receives the optimum of all nutrients it needs for maturing and growing in the womb. These can vary, depending on the phase of pregnancy the woman is currently in. Here it is now important to find a balanced average of nutrients to meet the needs of mother and child equally.

The emphasis here is on "balanced". There is often still the misconception that women who are pregnant have to eat for two people for the next nine months, i.e. they have "permission" to eat twice the amount of food. But this is by no means the case! Rampant eating is actually rather out of place and can even have a negative effect on your health and that of your child. The motto is rather: Do not **eat** for 2, but **think** for 2! By "thinking" we mean a responsible approach to nutrition. With it you have a very decisive lever in your hand to give your child a healthy start in life.

Important: Do not eat for 2, but think for 2!

With a balanced, healthy and varied diet, the focus is primarily on quality rather than quantity. Many women do not know at the beginning that the energy requirement and consequently the number of kilocalories (kcal) increases noticeably only in the second half of the pregnancy. This is when the baby starts to grow properly and consequently gains weight. Which brings us to the next point: weight gain!

During a normal pregnancy, the weight of the mother-to-be increases by 10 to 14 kilograms. On the one hand, this is of course due to the weight of the child, but the blood volume has also increased, the amniotic fluid, the placenta, and the increase in the tissue of the uterus and breasts naturally weigh a lot.

The energy requirement during pregnancy per day increases by 250-300 kcal compared to the requirement outside of pregnancy. That is not very much, if you consider that 100 grams of wholemeal bread already contain almost 300 kcal.
In the first two thirds of pregnancy, the woman's weight gain increases by about 300 grams per week; in the last third it is about 500 grams per week.

Important: Quality instead of quantity!

Much more important than the amount of food, are now the nutrients that are supplied to the body. The child will get what it needs from the mother. Achieving a balanced ratio here is essential to promote the healthy development of the baby. Considering that the woman's body is performing at its best, it is extremely important to supply it with all the nutrients it needs to help it develop its new life. After all, it is now necessary to develop a completely new human being: Heart, liver, kidneys and co, nerves, brain and eyes... All of this must have matured to a certain degree within a few months, so that the little person can see the light of day in good health.

Even if you are one of those women who have struggled with your weight from time to time throughout your life, a weight-reducing diet during pregnancy should be an absolute taboo. Now it is not a matter of taking nutrients away from the body, but rather of giving it the right ones in an appropriate amount.

But what exactly is important in detail when talking about a balanced diet? Which nutrients should you pay attention to exactly, how/ with what can you take them in and what should you perhaps even avoid? Allowed is allowed, what tastes good is a great saying, but especially during pregnancy there are indeed foods that can transmit pathogens and can endanger your and your baby's health considerably.
If you follow some "rules of conduct", however, you can avoid these dangers very well. Before we turn our attention to this topic, I would like to give you an overview of the nutrients in nutrition. This knowledge will help you to better understand some of the interrelationships.
So, let us now dive into the secret world of nutrients!

The secret world of nutrients

You have probably heard the term "nutrients" many times before. Even in this book we have used it several times. But what exactly does it actually mean? Which substances are affected by it and where are they everywhere? And even more important: Which ones should you pay particular attention to during your pregnancy and how can you best consume them?

If we look at the definition once, a "nutrient" is no more (but also no less) than a substance on which organisms can feed.

This affects organic and inorganic substances that are necessary and important for the way of life of people to generate energy in the body. Nutrients are absorbed through food and then metabolized in the organism through complex processes. In this way, all substances reach exactly those body parts and cells where they are needed. Quite cleverly thought up by Mother Nature, isn't it?

Nutrients can be divided into the subcategory's carbohydrates, proteins, fats, trace elements / minerals and vitamins. What now belongs to what and where they are hidden everywhere, you ask yourself? This is exactly what we will take a closer look at in detail.

Carbohydrates

Carbohydrates are the "fuel" of our organism and support our muscle and brain work. This is no different during pregnancy. Right now, your child needs carbohydrates to grow and mature. However, you should make sure that the daily portion of carbohydrates is not too large in the long term, as this can cause your baby to grow very quickly and as a result become very large. This in turn can have negative health effects for both of you.

A distinction is made between low- and high-quality carbohydrates.
Inferior carbohydrates are found, for example, in household or fruit sugar. If we consume these sugars, they enter the bloodstream immediately and are thus available to our organism very quickly. A separate splitting of the sugar is not necessary. The blood sugar rises immediately and

provides a small, short-term energy boost and the small sagging, which one just had, is thus quickly passé.

However, this energetic upswing does not last long, and foods with simple carbohydrates do not fill up for long either. On the contrary: the blood sugar level drops rapidly again after some time, which is noticeable by an attack of ravenous appetite and a renewed desire for sweets.

White household sugar not only has a negative effect on the bacteria in our intestinal flora, it also does not provide any vitamins and minerals, which are very important for a functioning digestion. In fact, these are "empty" carbohydrates that you supply to your body.

On the other hand, it makes much more sense to consume more of the "good" carbohydrates.

However, these must first be broken down into separate sugar building blocks by the body piece by piece after the intake of food. Only then can they be further utilized.

This has the great advantage that we feel fuller for longer. And this is independent of whether a pregnancy exists or not.

That's why it definitely makes sense to consume carbohydrates of the highest possible quality. These are found, for example, in **pulses**, **fruit**, **vegetables** and **cereals**. In addition to sugar, the body also gets a good portion of important vitamins, minerals and trace elements, which are vital for a healthy organism.

In the meantime, there are a number of sugar and sweetening variants on the market that are intended to replace household sugar.

Sweetener, for example, is a food additive, has no nutritional value whatsoever and is excreted by the body unchanged.

Sugar substitutes can be found in sugar-free drinks and foods, and they listen to the unpronounceable name's cyclamate, aspartame, acesulfame, neohesperidine or saccharin. They have an extremely intense sweet taste and, if consumed in moderation, do not harm pregnancy.

However, the consumption of sugar substitutes, such as mannitol, isomalt, xylitol, sorbitol, maltitol and lactitol, should be taken with caution.
They cannot be completely absorbed by the small intestine and therefore reach the large intestine virtually unchanged. There, these substances bind water and, if consumed in excess, can lead to diarrhea, flatulence and abdominal cramps. In the worst case, this can even trigger contractions.

If all these sweeteners are not really recommendable, what do you have left? Don't worry, you won't have to do without sweets during your pregnancy!

If you are one of those women who have a particular weakness for sweet foods, then it is best to leave white household sugar & the other alternatives mentioned above to one side and prefer to use sweeteners such as agave syrup, maple syrup, raw cane sugar, mascobado or primal sweetness (dried sugar juice) during your pregnancy.

Proteins (proteins)

Especially during pregnancy your body has an increased need for protein to support the growth of your child.

Proteins, also known as proteins, are the building blocks of every cell and therefore an indispensable component of a healthy diet.

If you eat a varied and balanced diet, you can easily reach the necessary amount (from the 4th month approx. 60 grams daily) without much effort.

Proteins fill you up for a long time, keep your blood sugar level stable and thus reduce the danger of ravenous attacks on sweets. Thus, proteins are an optimal way to save kilocalories.

Protein can be found in milk, dairy products, fish, eggs, meat and cereals, for example. Here it is particularly important that you consume foods that have a particularly high biological value. It describes how much of the food protein can be converted into body protein. The higher this value is, the more valuable a protein is.

The above-mentioned foods already have this high value. Please also note, however, that you should not throw yourself uncontrollably into meat and sausage products. Especially in you there are often hidden fats that are anything but good for you. This also applies to cheese products. These can also be a real little "fat bomb". If you are among those who have to keep an eye on your weight, it is advisable to fall back on the low-fat or low-fat variants.

Only with fish products is a high fat content even beneficial to the health of your baby. In fact, the following applies here: the fatter, the better! Fat-rich fish such as mackerel, salmon and herring provide you with essential fatty acids and iodine, which in turn is extremely important for your thyroid gland (more on this later).

If you succeed in achieving a balanced average between vegetable and animal protein suppliers, you will have a top protein quality! Therefore, you should preferably choose vegetable foods, such as pulses, whole meal products or nuts, and flank them with yoghurt, milk, curd cheese, lean cheese, etc.

You can easily meet your daily protein requirements with three small portions of milk or dairy products. For example, 1 glass of milk, 1 cup of yoghurt and 1 slice of whole meal bread with cheese already covers some of your protein requirements.

In addition, you can also treat yourself to fatty sea fish 2 times a week and 3-4 portions of lean meat.

Greases

One thing in advance: Fats are healthy - **if** they are the right ones!

Fats contain twice as many calories as carbohydrates and proteins and are the most important energy stores in our body and therefore essential for survival. That is why fats should never be avoided.
This is no different during pregnancy. If the nutritional requirements change in many areas, the fat requirement is not particularly increased in this special phase.
A fat content of 25-30 percent (equivalent to approx. 80 grams) per day is perfectly sufficient.

Fatty acids cannot be produced by the body itself. They must therefore be supplied to the organism with food from outside. It is important that you make sure that a good mixture of animal and vegetable fats is produced when putting the fats together.

In this context, the reference to hidden fats is also permitted. These lurk in many finished products, sausage and cheese varieties, desserts and pastries. A very moderate approach is really required here. For meat and sausage products, it is better to use lean meat (e.g. chicken/turkey breast or steak).

While you may be a little more generous, the consumption of nuts and seeds, olives, avocado, but also various virgin, cold-pressed oils (egg, olive, diesel, sunflower or canola oil). They all provide you with valuable, polyunsaturated fatty acids and vitamins A and E. Animal fats on the other hand contain Vitamin D and lecithin.

When using oils, please also pay attention to which of them are suitable for cooking and frying. Refined oils (e.g. olive oil, rapeseed oil, sunflower oil) are more suitable for braising, steaming and short frying.
Cold pressed oils, on the other hand, are more suitable for the cold kitchen. Use them to enrich your salad or season your pasta or vegetables. They are particularly tasty and are therefore best suited for dishes of this kind.

Oils of any kind should always be stored in a cool and dark place (preferably in the refrigerator). This is the only way to preserve the healthy fatty acids. Opened bottles should be used up within 4 to 8 weeks if possible.

At this point I would like to emphasize once again the omega-3 fatty acids. They are true multi-talents!
They are extremely important not only during pregnancy, but also during lactation, as they are needed for the healthy development of the brain and eyes. Pregnant women should consume at least 200 mg omega-3 fatty acids per day. These can be found especially in fatty fish (I already mentioned examples above).

If you do not like fish, you can also take fish oil capsules. However, you should consult your doctor before doing so. He will advise you about certain preparations and the individual amount required.
You can also use more rape, walnut and linseed oil in the kitchen. They contain a precursor of these important fatty acids, which in turn are then converted in the body into the coveted omega-3 fatty acids.

Trace elements & minerals

Trace elements and minerals are inorganic nutrients and can be found in both animal and vegetable food. Humans need only very small quantities of them and yet a deficiency of them can lead to complaints or developmental disorders in the unborn child.

In order to give you a short overview, I will list the most important trace elements and minerals in the following.

Calcium:

Calcium is extremely important for tooth and bone formation, but also for the development of your baby's muscles and nerves. Your baby gets what he or she needs, if necessary, from your reserves. Especially in the case of a lack of calcium, this can lead to an increased risk of osteoporosis if you do not take in sufficient amounts of this trace element through your diet. In addition, it can also lead to pre-eclampsia (high blood pressure during pregnancy) and muscle cramps during pregnancy.

Calcium is particularly effective when combined with vitamins C, K and D, as well as magnesium.

Food sources of calcium: milk, yogurt, cheese, almonds, broccoli, spinach, peas, beans, cabbage

Iron:

Iron is essential for the development of muscles and the formation of red blood cells. During pregnancy, the body needs about 3 milligrams of iron per day, almost twice as much as usual. If the iron requirement is not covered on a long-term basis, this can even lead to anemia (lack of blood) and an increased risk of premature birth.

Iron can be absorbed by the body particularly well in combination with Vitamin C.

Food sources of iron: red meat, broccoli, spinach, peas, whole grains, legumes, cabbage, seafood, sunflower seeds, strawberries, beetroot (-juice)

Copper:

This trace element is essential for the formation of the heart and the circulatory system of your child. Particularly in the last trimester, a lot of copper is needed when the metabolic functions of the heart and the immune system are running at full speed.

Food sources for copper: spinach, beetroot, beans, whole grain products, hazelnuts, peas, asparagus, quinoa

Magnesium:

Magnesium is a real multi-talent: healthy bones & cells, blood clotting, lowering high blood pressure, alleviating calf cramps, migraines and sleep disorders - all this is due to a sufficient magnesium supply. It also promotes the absorption of calcium and can reduce morning sickness. A lower rate of miscarriages and premature births is another important aspect that illustrates the importance of a sufficient magnesium intake.

Food sources of copper: sunflower and pumpkin seeds, broccoli, spinach, beetroot, peas, beans, whole grain products, milk

Zinc:

This mineral also has a significant influence on the development of your child's bones and nervous system. If the expectant mother does not have enough zinc, the risk of neural tube damage and low birth weight increases.

Food sources for zinc: Red meat, whole grain products, poultry, pumpkin seeds

Selenium:

Selenium is a highly effective antioxidant, which is particularly important for cell development. If the body has too little available, the risk of miscarriage and pre-eclampsia increases.

Food sources for selenium: Almonds, walnuts, whole meal products, fish, poultry, eggs, garlic, red meat

Potassium:

Potassium is a mineral, which is essential for a balanced electrolyte balance as well as for energy supply, muscle and nerve impulses and the increase of blood volume. If you suffer more frequently from calf cramps, an increased intake of potassium can be helpful.

Food sources of potassium: beetroot, beans, fish, lentils, potatoes, figs, avocados, yogurt, bananas

Manganese:

This is a mineral which is important for the formation of strong bones. Especially in combination with copper it protects against cell damage and promotes energy production.

Food sources for manganese: Lentils, hazelnuts, almonds, kale, spinach, beans, raspberries, whole grain products

Chrome:

Chromium is a trace element which ensures that proteins are formed in the child's tissue. If you suffer from diabetes, or currently suffer from pregnancy diabetes, chromium is particularly important because it regulates the blood sugar level.

Food sources for chromium: poultry, eggs, spinach, lettuce, bananas, apples, beef

Phosphorus:

This mineral works particularly well with calcium. It has a particular effect on the formation of healthy bones and teeth - both for you and your child.
Phosphorus also has a great influence on the smooth functioning of nerves, heart, kidneys and muscles and regulates energy consumption.

Food sources of phosphorus: milk, cheese, yogurt, eggs, lentils, peas, beans, fish, poultry

Iodine:

Iodine is particularly important for the function of your child's thyroid gland. A lack of iodine can lead to disorders in the mental and physical development of the child. The recommended amount of iodine that should be taken in addition to the daily intake is between 100 and 150 micrograms. If necessary, the intake of iodine tablets is recommended. However, you should discuss this with your doctor in advance, especially if there is a thyroid dysfunction.

Food sources for iodine: sea fish, dairy products, iodine-containing table salt

All minerals and trace elements are listed here once again with the recommended daily amount during pregnancy:

Nutrient	Recommended daily amount	Food
Calcium	1,2 g	milk, yogurt, cheese, almonds, broccoli, spinach, peas, beans, cabbage
Iron	3 mg	red meat, broccoli, spinach, peas, wholemeal products, legumes, cabbage, seafood, sunflower seeds, strawberries, beetroot (-juice)
Copper	1 mg	Spinach, beetroot, beans, wholemeal products, hazelnuts, peas, asparagus, quinoa
Magnesium	310 mg	Sunflower and pumpkin seeds, broccoli, spinach, beetroot, peas, bean, wholemeal products, milk, oat flakes, amaranth

Zinc	10 mg	meat, wholemeal products, poultry, pumpkin seeds, flaxseed, oat flakes
Selenium	60-70mcg	Almonds, walnuts, wholemeal products, fish, poultry, eggs, garlic, red meat
Potassium	4000mg	beet, beans, fish, lentils, potatoes, figs, avocados, yogurt, bananas
Manganese	2.5- 5.0 mg	Lentils, hazelnuts, almonds, kale, spinach, beans, raspberries, whole grain products
Chrome	30-100 mcg	poultry, eggs, spinach, lettuce, bananas, apples, beef
phosphorus	800 mg	milk, cheese, yogurt, eggs, lentils, peas, beans, fish, poultry
Iodine	200-230 mcg	sea fish, dairy products, iodized table salt

So much for the topic trace elements. Quite extensive, isn't it? And this is "only" a rough overview of which of them are important for you during pregnancy. But that is not enough. The best possible supply of trace elements and minerals is not the only thing you should pay attention to.

A very special importance is also attached to various vitamins, which we will now take a closer look at in detail.

Vitamins

Vitamins are healthy - that much is certain!
They ensure that muscles, bones and our immune system are strengthened. In addition, they also have an influence on our digestion and help to build up skin and other tissue.
Vitamins are therefore vital nutrients, which our body cannot produce itself in most cases. We have to help here and supply them to the body from outside, for example with food.

At this point I would like to concentrate on the vitamins that are especially important for you and your child during pregnancy. During this time, your need for some vitamins will also be increased.
If the needs outside a pregnancy are still well covered by a balanced diet, it is indeed necessary to take some vitamins in tablet form during pregnancy. I will explain which exactly these are in the following.

Vitamin A:

A low Vitamin A level weakens the immune system and increases susceptibility to infection. Vitamin A is very important for intensive cell growth and thus for the maturation of the baby. The eyes and the liver are especially supported by Vitamin A. Especially in the second and last third of the pregnancy, care should be taken to ensure a sufficient supply. Please note that an excess of this Vitamin can lead to damage in the development of the fetus.

Food sources of Vitamin A: butter, eggs, cheese, fatty fish, beetroot, peas, broccoli, asparagus, pumpkin, carrots, spinach

B Vitamins:

The B vitamins are composed of 8 water-soluble vitamins in total. These are B1 (thiamine), B2 (riboflavin), B3 (niacin), B5 (pantothenic acid), B6 (pyridoxine), B7 (biotin), B9 (folic acid) and B12 (cobalamin).

You have certainly come across one or the other in the form of a different name. Biotin and folic acid are certainly familiar to you.

But did you know that vitamins B1, B2 and B3 are responsible for the development of the baby's nervous system, brain or muscles? Whereas B6 and B12 regulate the stress hormones and promote stamina.

A sufficient amount of B vitamins is therefore vital for the healthy development of your child.

During pregnancy you have an increased need for B1 and B2. With them you replenish your energy stores, ensure a functioning nerve and muscle activity and promote iron absorption.

Regular use of B6 can help reduce nausea. A B12 preparation might be useful for vegetarians or vegans to prevent neurological damage to the unborn child.

Food sources for B vitamins: eggs, milk, yogurt, red meat, sunflower seeds, hard cheese, almonds, wholemeal products, avocados, almonds

Folic acid (folate):

This Vitamin has already appeared above in the B vitamins (B9). However, it is considered to be of such importance that I would like to list it separately at this point.

Foliature is the central B Vitamin not only *in,* but also already *before* a pregnancy. But what makes this Vitamin so special?

Folic acid contributes significantly to reducing the risk of damage to the neural tube (e.g. spina bifida = open back). It promotes the formation of red blood cells and DNA. You should now take an amount of 400 micrograms daily in addition to your normal diet. Please discuss the choice of a suitable preparation with your doctor.

This Vitamin is found more often in green vegetables, whole grain products and legumes. However, it is difficult to cover the increased need for folic acid with meals alone. Therefore, you should definitely help here in the form of dietary supplements. Basically, the intake of folic acid should be started before pregnancy so that a sufficient amount of this Vitamin is available in the body early enough.

Food sources of folic acid: beetroot, broccoli, spinach, peas, asparagus, pumpkin, beans, blackberries, avocados, chickpeas, whole grain products, eggs, bananas, pomegranates

Vitamin C:

Just about everyone knows that Vitamin C is healthy and strengthens our immune system. But did you know that it also contributes to the formation of new tissue and promotes the absorption of iron? If your Vitamin C budget is covered, you will prevent gum bleeding and nausea during pregnancy and also reduce the risk of preeclampsia.

Food sources of Vitamin C: oranges, strawberries, kiwi, grapefruit, blackberries, raspberries, Brussels sprouts, broccoli, tomatoes, spinach, pumpkin, kale, peppers, peas, asparagus

Vitamin D:

This Vitamin is essential for your baby's well-developed and strong bones and teeth, but it is also extremely important for your own bones and teeth to have your Vitamin D needs met. But not only that! Vitamin D also contributes significantly to an active immune system and strong muscles and protects the nerve cells of the brain.

Since Vitamin D is produced in the skin, you can actually cover your need for it very easily through sunlight. A daily stay outside in daylight, for example by going for a walk, can be sufficient. You should make sure that the sun's rays have unhindered access to your skin and that it is not covered by clothing. If this is not possible for you, please discuss with your doctor whether it is advisable to take a supplement under certain circumstances.
Adults, regardless of pregnancy, should take 20 micrograms daily.

Food sources of Vitamin D: broccoli, spinach, Brussels sprouts, kale, lettuce, asparagus

Vitamin K:

Vitamin K also contributes to healthy and strong bones and can also reduce morning sickness and promote blood clotting.

Food sources of Vitamin K: Spinach, Brussels sprouts, broccoli, asparagus, kale

Here too, all vitamins are clearly displayed once again:

Vitamin	Recommended daily amount	Food
Vitamin A	1.1 mg	butter, eggs, cheese, fatty fish, beetroot, peas, broccoli, asparagus, pumpkin, carrots, spinach
Vitamin B1 (thiamine)	1.2 mg	wholemeal products, oat flakes, green peas
Vitamin B2 (riboflavin)	1.5 mg	almonds, yeast flakes, mushrooms, peas
Vitamin B3 (niacin)	14-16 mg	meat, fish, dairy products, poultry, eggs
Vitamin B5 (pantothenic acid)	6 mg	Red meat, milk, eggs, fish, oatmeal, wholemeal products, avocado, broccoli, legumes
Vitamin B6 (pyridoxine)	1.5 - 1.8 mg	potatoes, avocado, nuts, fish, dairy products, poultry
Vitamin B7 (biotin)	30 - 60 µg*	liver, eggs, nuts, oatmeal, cheese

Vitamin B9 (folic acid)	550 µg*	Tomatoes, asparagus, wholemeal products, eggs, salad, broccoli, spinach, peas
Vitamin B12 (cobalamin)	4.5 µg*	meat, fish, seafood, dairy products, eggs
Vitamin C	95 mg	oranges, strawberries, kiwi, grapefruit, blackberries, raspberries, Brussels sprouts, broccoli, tomatoes, spinach, pumpkin, kale, peppers, peas, asparagus
Vitamin D	20 µg*	broccoli, spinach, Brussels sprouts, kale, lettuce, asparagus
Vitamin K	60 µg*	spinach, Brussels sprouts, broccoli, asparagus, kale

*µg=microgram

So much for the most important vitamins that are relevant for you during your pregnancy. Sounds pretty complex? It is! But once you have familiarized yourself a little bit with the subject, you will surely not find it so difficult to pay attention to the beneficial foods and to achieve a healthy mixture.

Have you noticed that a lot of foods keep popping up? Spinach, broccoli, peas, asparagus, beans, yogurt and beetroot are just some of them, which are rich in vitamins as well as minerals and trace elements. If you follow these common foods and include them in your meals more often, you will already be providing yourself with several of these essential vitamins and trace elements each time.

Do you feel a little overwhelmed by all the theoretical knowledge and you don't have a brilliant idea how to integrate all this into your everyday life? Don't worry, it is not that difficult! That's exactly why we have listed numerous recipes in this guide to help you get started with this extensive topic.

All dishes are easy and quick to prepare, taste delicious and accompany you reliably every day on your way to a balanced and varied diet.

Whether it's main meals, a small snack in between, refreshing drinks or even a delicious smoothie - you're sure to find something to your taste. Be curious!

What you should avoid now!

On the last few pages we have looked in detail at everything that you should eat during your pregnancy in sufficient quantities and in increased quantities.

However, there are also some things to consider that should be avoided at all costs, as they can be extremely dangerous for your and/or your child's health. What exactly is affected, you may ask? This is exactly what this chapter is about.

Avoid raw products!
As a rule of thumb, the expectant mother should avoid all raw foods for the duration of the pregnancy. This includes raw meat, raw eggs, raw milk products and raw fish. But why exactly? What is the danger?

Quite simply, untreated, raw foods are at increased risk of contracting a wide variety of infections.

Raw eggs and raw poultry may be infected with salmonella. These in turn can lead to severe diarrhea and, under certain circumstances, to premature labor.

In eggs and egg dishes, on the other hand, which are cooked and poultry, which is sufficiently fried, the salmonella are killed by the heating process. A safe consumption of these foods is therefore only guaranteed by this preparation method.

Another very important factor is the increased risk of infection with Listeria. No, this does not mean the mouthwash for gargling.

These are rather bacteria that can be found in milk, dairy products, fish, meat, soft cheese, but also in pre-cut salads. They cause the so-called listeriosis.

Even if, fortunately, infection with Listeria is rare, you should play it safe during pregnancy and avoid eating these foods in raw form. After all, an infection can lead to serious health problems for the unborn child. Even if the pregnant woman has "only" flu-like symptoms (if at all), the baby can suffer considerable damage. The bacterium is very resistant and multiplies even at refrigerator temperatures. Even a visit to the freezer will not harm them. Only heating these foods to at least 70 degrees kills them reliably. That's why you should always choose pasteurized versions for dairy products. You can consume these without hesitation.

Another important source of infection is toxoplasmosis. This is a parasitic risk of infection, which can be transmitted to humans through raw meat or cat excrement. This also includes soil, sand, grass, etc. contaminated by cat excrement.

If a woman becomes infected with the toxoplasmosis pathogen for the first-time during pregnancy, this can lead to transmission to the baby and cause severe deformities, disabilities and even miscarriages.

If you are not sure whether you are immune to this pathogen, you can easily find out by a blood test with your doctor.

For the safest possible protection, you should therefore consistently avoid eating raw meat and (if you have a house cat at home) clean the litter box only with high hygienic measures.

Since the pathogen can also spread outside "in the countryside", you should always wash fruit, vegetables and salad extremely thoroughly before consumption.

In the following I will briefly and concisely list what you can do yourself to avoid food infections:

- Wash your hands thoroughly on a regular basis.
- Leftover food, meat, fish and eggs should be kept in the refrigerator be stored.
- Make sure that the cold chain is uninterrupted for these foods.
- Raw food should be stored separately in order to avoid the transmission of pathogens.
- Frozen foods are best defrosted in the refrigerator early.
- Vegetables and fruit are very thorough (!) before consumption under cold Water off to wash.
- Cook or fry fish and meat well on all sides; the core temperature should be at least 70 degrees.
- Avoid the consumption of raw milk, raw milk products and raw egg dishes
- The same applies to raw meat and raw fish.

Apart from food, hygiene is now the be-all and end-all! It is best to change dishcloths and dish towels every day, work surfaces should be cleaned with hot water and for food preparation you should use separate work boards for meat, fish, poultry, vegetables & Co.

That was a lot of theory on one swing. So that you now know exactly which foods you should avoid during your pregnancy, I have listed them here:

Meat	minced meat, tartar, carpaccio, raw sausage (salami, mead sausage, tea sausage, liver sausage, Parma ham), offal
Fish	Sushi, smoked and marinated fish products, herring salad
Vegetables	Avoid pre-cut and packaged salad mixes, sprouts, rolls or sandwiches topped with lettuce/tomato/cucumber
Fruit	Unwashed fruit or products thereof, e.g. freshly squeezed juice at juice counters
Raw milk products	Camembert, Brie, Ricotta, Feta
Raw eggs	Tiramisu, homemade mayonnaise, raw cake dough
Spices (in large quantities)	thyme, marjoram, cloves, cinnamon, ginger, cardamom

Finally, to this chapter, I want to mention two things, which should be self-evident, but which I want to mention again for the sake of completeness.

Both alcohol and nicotine should be avoided completely during pregnancy. Both are pure poison, which is supplied directly to the unborn child via the umbilical cord, and later also to the baby via breast milk.

In the womb, alcohol can lead to malformations of the heart, kidneys and limbs, as well as to mental retardation. Remember that alcohol is also contained in various sweet things (e.g. chocolates or tiramisu). In the latter not only alcohol but also raw egg is processed.

When choosing your drinks, please note that you should be sparing with caffeinated liquids. You do not have to do without coffee and black tea completely, but you should limit your consumption to 3 cups a day. The caffeine enters the baby's bloodstream via the placenta and can lead to an increased heartbeat in the unborn child.

You should also avoid energy drinks altogether, as they contain even more caffeine than coffee or tea.

Bitter Lemon and Tonic Water are also drinks which are not without danger for the child due to their quinine content. Towards the end of pregnancy, they can even trigger premature contractions. It is also best to refrain from them for the duration of the pregnancy.

Optimal nutrition in the 1st trimester

The first 3 months of pregnancy (4th to 13th week of pregnancy): What an exciting time in a woman's life! Two tiny little cells that have made themselves comfortable in your uterus will turn your life upside down in the near future. Now many expectant mothers ask themselves what they are allowed, should or even have to eat at all during this special time.

In this early phase of pregnancy, the hormones change, which is often accompanied by unpleasant side effects for the pregnant woman such as morning sickness, tiredness, constipation, ravenous appetite attacks and heartburn.
Towards the end of the first trimester, the small embryo is already recognizable as a complete small human being, even if with about 7.5 cm still quite tiny.
And yet, both your baby and yourself need special care and attention now. In addition to sufficient rest and relaxation, it is now important that your body receives all the important nutrients for a good development of your child. A well-balanced mixed diet will help you to achieve this.

Special attention should now be paid to the increase of folic acid (folate), Vitamin A and iron.
High suppliers of these nutrients are for example spinach, peas, kale and broccoli. There are numerous tasty recipes that you can use to cover your needs for the nutrients you

need in a delicious and easy way. The recipes in this book will certainly help you to find inspiration and to try them out.

If you are hungry for something sweet, you may also become weak at times. However, you should consider it an exception and leave it at one portion. It is better to take an extra portion of fruit as a snack between meals. A handful of berries not only satisfies your hunger for something sweet, but also provides you and your little one with important nutrients and vitamins. Tastes good and does good! What more do we want?!

If you feel that you cannot eat solid food because of morning sickness, the smoothies & drinks in this book may be a good alternative for you. Just give it a try!

Do you also pack cravings for the classic "Pickles & Chocolate" in between? No fear! This is not unusual. The hormones are to blame for this, which can cause a lot of trouble in a woman's body, especially in the early stages of pregnancy. During this exciting time, the sense of taste and smell also changes, which can sometimes lead to the fact that some smells trigger a spontaneous nausea, while others suddenly make your mouth water. All this is normal and disappears again at the latest after the birth of the child.

Optimal nutrition in the second trimester

The second trimester ranges from the 14th SSW to the 27th SSW and now also shows the first signs of pregnancy on the outside. The unpleasant side effects from the 1st trimester slowly subside. However, the baby's belly now increases in size, which naturally leads to an increase in the belly circumference of the expectant mother. The clothes, which fitted without any problems a few weeks ago, are now tightening more and more and the breasts are also gaining volume. This means that the woman's body is already preparing for breastfeeding later.

He is now building up reserves, which is why he needs a complete and vital substance-rich diet during this time. The following nutrients are needed in this phase by both the mother and the child:

Folic acid, calcium, iodine, selenium, omega-3 fatty acids, iron, vitamins B6 & B12, Vitamin C.

The average energy requirement increases in the 2nd trimester to about 250 kcal per day. That is about 1 apple and 0.5 L of buttermilk additionally. As you can see, even if the unborn child now rapidly increases in size and weight, this has only a very slight effect on the amount of food you eat. As mentioned above, it is actually the nutrient and energy balance of individual foods that counts more than the quantity as such.

> **Important: Do not eat twice as much, but eat twice as well!**

Optimal nutrition in the third trimester

From the 28th SSW the third and last trimester begins. This is the most stressful time for the pregnant woman, because during this time she literally has to carry the "load" in the form of the additional weight. Once this phase has been reached, the body needs an additional 250 kcal every day.

The child is constantly growing in size and the space in the belly is becoming less and less. You should now eat smaller meals more frequently. Five small meals can now be eaten better than three large ones, for which at a certain point there is simply not enough space in the abdomen.
What your body now needs more of is dietary fiber, Vitamin K, Vitamin C and Vitamin B1.
Now reach boldly into the fruit basket and allow yourself an extra shot of Vitamin C from time to time. It not only helps your body to strengthen the immune system, but also ensures that the iron in your diet can be better absorbed.

Regardless of which stage of pregnancy you are at, you should always ensure that you have a sufficient fluid intake. You should drink 2-3 liters of magnesium-containing mineral water or tap water daily. If you suffer from heartburn frequently, still water is probably best for you.

Important: Drink 2-3 liters of fluid daily.

Vegetarians and Vegans: A little "extra sausage

How complex the nutrition during pregnancy is, we have discussed in detail on the last pages. But how does this actually apply to women who avoid animal products or only ingest them in very small amounts?

Vegetarians as well as Vegan have at least already times the advantage that you can skip everything approximately around the raw meat in its most multicolored prescription facets confidently. But are women, who only take certain, and/or no animal products to itself, on the safe side, if of a balanced nutrition the speech is the answer is a very clear "yes"!

Women who categorically exclude animal products altogether (vegans) are very unlikely to have the required amount of nutrients. Elementary components, such as iodine, zinc, omega-3 fatty acids, calcium, iron and vitamins B12, B2 and D are not supplied at all or only in very small quantities. The possibility of a nutrient deficiency due to an undersupply is actually quite given here.

If women would like to do now in addition, during the pregnancy without animal products completely, it is advisable to consult a nourishing consultation. There are qualified advisors, who specialized in vegetarian/vegan nutrition. With them it can be coordinated once exactly, how a nourishing nutrition can be achieved also without animal food. It is also of particular advantage that in a direct consultation the personal preferences and eating habits of the woman can be incorporated. Now we can look for an individual solution together.

Whether dietary supplements are appropriate under certain circumstances should be discussed with the treating physician. Regular blood tests during pregnancy reveal a nutrient deficiency at an early stage and allow for a quick adjustment of the diet.

Critical voices are often heard regarding vegan nutrition during pregnancy. This can also have positive effects. Often the blood sugar level is more stable with vegetarian, heartburn and constipation are less frequent and altogether less sugar is consumed, which again also benefits the teeth.

So pregnant and vegan can work well - if it is planned sensibly and the changed nutrient need is considered.

With vegetarians the lack of nutrients is not quite so extreme opposite the vegetarian. Women who also consume dairy products usually have no problems with deficiency symptoms.

Often, however, meat and fish are dispensed with, whereas the consumption of eggs and honey is allowed. This form of nutrition is called "ovo-lacto-vegetarian" nutrition and should generally ensure a sufficient supply of all-important nutrients and minerals. However, iodine, folic acid and omega-3 fatty acids (DHA) are exceptions to this rule.

The iron value should also be critically checked, as iron is found mainly in fish and meat.

In order to have certainty, it is advisable to talk to the doctor and, if necessary, check the values by means of a blood test.

Deficiency symptoms can thus be detected and specifically remedied by dietary supplements.

Problems during pregnancy

In hardly any other phase of life is the body of a woman exposed to such extremes.

Within 40 weeks, two small cells turn into a finished, viable human being. During this time, the woman's body runs at full speed, culminating in a true tour de force, the birth.

It is probably obvious to most women that not everything can go smoothly and without complications during these months.

And this does not only mean the pregnancy-related side effects such as nausea, tiredness or digestive problems. These, and many other possible complaints, we will look at in this chapter.

Heartburn

Especially in the 2nd and 3rd trimester this can be a very unpleasant side effect.

Due to the hormonal changes in the body, the tension in the stomach decreases slightly. As a result, the so-called "stomach gate muscle" sits somewhat looser. However, this makes it easier for the stomach contents to flow back into the esophagus, which can lead to the acidic belching, nausea and heartburn.

Even a too copious meal or a kick from the child can cause gastric juice to flow back into the esophagus.

That helps:

-Eat several small meals throughout the day rather than a few large ones.

-It is best to avoid greasy, fried, spicy, sour or spicy foods.

-Permit yourself a little moderate exercise after dinner, e.g. in the form of a walk.

-If you suffer acutely from heartburn, 2-3 tonsils may already help you. Chew them well until a real mush has formed in your mouth.   If you now swallow it, it binds the stomach acid.

- Drink a glass of cold milk or chew a rusk.

- Against nightly heartburn it can already help if you use elevated upper body sleep and the last meal before 6 pm take.

Back pain

Back pain is a complaint that occurs more often, especially in the second half of pregnancy.

The weight that the woman now has to carry is also noticeable in her posture. Due to the constantly increasing belly circumference, many pregnant women unconsciously end up with a hollow back. The back muscles are now increasingly strained by the rising weight. It is not uncommon for blockages to occur in the sacroiliac joint or, even more uncomfortable, for the child to press painfully on the sciatic nerve.

That helps:

- Go swimming more often. In the water your body has no weight to carry and you can make moderate movements quasi "weightless" and escape the whirlpool of pain and tension for a short time.

- If you suffer acutely from back pain, allow yourself some bed rest for a short time and place a grain pillow or a hot water bottle on the painful area.

- You should now avoid high shoes and fall back on flat shoes.

- Moderate gymnastic exercises may be able to help you many times. The following exercise you can simply do quietly from time to time:

Move into the four-footed position, form now - vertebra by vertebra - your spine into a "cat's hump"; breathe in and out deeply 1-2 times; release the cat's hump now vertebra by vertebra and come into a guided hollow back.

You can perform this sequence of movements 5-10 times in a row. It is important that you do it carefully and slowly. This is primarily about mobilizing and strengthening your spine and not about sporting ambitions.

Gestational Diabetes

Gestational diabetes, also known as gestational diabetes, is a metabolic disease that occurs mainly from the 24th week of pregnancy and affects about 8% of all pregnant women.

Often overweight women and those with a family history of diabetes are affected by this form of the disease.

This variant of "diabetes" often comes as a surprise to affected women, as it occurs unnoticed and silently. It often disappears again after pregnancy. What remains is the risk of developing diabetes mellitus type II in later years.

If women are told this diagnosis by their doctor, there is often understandably a great deal of uncertainty. If you already pay close attention to your diet during pregnancy, this is of course even more important with gestational diabetes.

"What does that mean for my baby?"; "What am I actually allowed to eat at all?"; "What do I have to pay attention to? "Am I not allowed to snack at all now," are just some of the questions frequently asked in this context. Don't worry! In the meantime, pregnancy diabetes can also be managed well, provided that the woman concerned follows a few rules.
A very important point is an appropriately adapted diet. There are now many suitable recipes that take diabetes into account and are still tasty and easy to prepare. Affected women therefore do not have to sacrifice taste or quality of life.

But what exactly does "diabetes" mean?
If diabetes is present, the body can no longer produce enough insulin to transport the carbohydrates (sugar) from the blood into the individual cells. The sugar now remains in the blood for too long. This can ultimately lead to the baby growing excessively and thus also to an increased birth weight. This, in turn, can lead to complications during pregnancy or birth. In addition, the risk of both mother and child becoming permanently ill with diabetes increases.

In order to avoid this, it is once again necessary to critically question one's own eating habits in the case of diagnosed gestational diabetes and to deal with it even more consciously. The good news is that with a change in diet and a little moderate exercise, the risks of the disease can already be significantly reduced.

You should now increase your consumption of salad and vegetables a little, because both contain a lot of water and fiber, which have no influence on blood sugar.

Note that carbohydrates and sugars are now also not completely prohibited. Today, we know that it should be the right carbohydrates that women consume and that sweets are not completely taboo.

That helps:
- Eat little sugar and white flour products.
- Prefer whole grain foods rich in fiber and fresh vegetables.
- Only eat fruit in moderation because of its fructose content (this includes especially fruit juices).
- Avoid synthetic sweeteners, such as acesulfame, cyclamate, saccharin.
- It is better to eat 6 small meals a day than 2-3 large ones.
- Avoid stress.

To take away any uncertainties, you should discuss the individual details with your doctor. He will give you helpful tips on how to behave best in your case, which foods to avoid and which type of sport or exercise is best for you.

Constipation

During pregnancy, the intestines often become somewhat sluggish, which leads to the feeling that you cannot empty yourself as you would like to.

What you should not do now is to take laxatives on your own. You should also not "push" to relieve yourself when you go to the toilet (you are allowed to do this enough during the birth). It's best to try it in a gentle way first using the options below and see how your body reacts.

That helps:
- psyllium husks, wheat bran and linseed in your yoghurt or mixed with your muesli, stimulates the intestinal activity.
- Eat figs, dried plums or apricots, whole meal products, sauerkraut, raw fruits and vegetables
- Make sure you get enough exercise in the fresh air; 30 Walking for a few minutes already has a positive effect on the intestinal activity off.
- Make sure that you drink enough liquid.

If this does not solve your digestive problem and/or if you suffer from pain during bowel movements, you should immediately discuss this with your doctor or midwife.

Calf Cramps

If you suffer from recurring calf cramps, this may be a sign of magnesium deficiency. It is not uncommon for this to cause you to wake up in the middle of the night in a very ungentle manner. This does not necessarily need to worry you, but it is still a signal from the body that you should check your magnesium intake and increase it slightly if necessary.

That helps:

- Eat food containing magnesium: whole meal products, milk and dairy products
   and lots of green vegetables.
- Drink mineral water containing magnesium.
- Every now and then, consciously treat yourself to a small "vein pump" and perform the following exercise:
To do this, stand alternately on your tiptoes and then on your heels. Now slowly and gently tap your feet a few times from your toes to your heels.
This easy and quick exercise supports blood circulation in the legs and can prevent calf cramps.

Nausea and vomiting

Unfortunately, for the majority of women, both are among the inevitable side effects of pregnancy. Many pregnant women have to struggle with morning sickness in the first weeks and months.

It can also happen that some of them are nauseous from morning to night, which can make this phase of the pregnancy a little difficult.

Most likely this nausea is caused by the pregnancy hormone HCG in the woman's body, which increases enormously, especially in the first three months. After the 12th week, this value drops again somewhat, which would also explain why the nausea often subsides then.

That helps:
- Get up slowly and gently from bed in the morning; abrupt movements can cause spontaneous nausea.
- Avoid fatty foods and feed yourself with fresh and nutritious food, spread over several small meals a day.

- Avoid finished products & fast food.
- Treat yourself to peace and quiet and relax now and then conscious; here small meditation units can be very helpful be.
- If you vomit frequently and strongly, dried fruit can be damaged by the contained potassium to compensate for the loss of electrolyte.
- If you suffer from persistent nausea, bitter substances from artichokes may be present, Grapefruit, radicchio and rocket salad help.

Tiredness

Increased fatigue during pregnancy is not uncommon and quite understandable. Your body is now performing at its absolute peak, which can also drain your energy reserves.

Listen to your body and allow yourself a little time out now and then, if necessary, even in broad daylight.

Also try to follow up your possibly increased need for sleep - your body needs this rest urgently. Similar to nausea, this symptom of tiredness often subsides after the first three months.

That helps:
- Put a small gentle gymnastic unit outdoors from time to time, or but at the opened window; this brings the circulation back into swing and you get an extra portion of oxygen
- Treat yourself to a drink every now and then during the day small snack in the form of nuts, a muesli bar, dried fruit or fresh fruit or vegetables
- You should now also avoid hard to digest, fatty and large

portions with your meals - these are the ones you are most comfortable with quite heavy in the stomach.
- Think about a sufficient fluid intake; the best thing is to at least two liters daily.

12 General tips

Having arrived at this point in the book, you have already learned a lot about what is important for a healthy, balanced diet during pregnancy. You now know what unpleasant side effects you might be confronted with and have perhaps already made the acquaintance of one or the other.

Apart from that, I would like to give you **12 tips** in this chapter that may be helpful for you not only during pregnancy but also during the breastfeeding period.

Tip 1: Don't let yourself be stressed - also and above all not while eating. You do not feel like cooking? Then leave it alone and treat yourself to a slice of wholegrain bread with lean sausage or cheese instead. Snack a few vegetable sticks and if you like, put your legs up in the process. Whatever is good for you is allowed.

Tip 2: Which brings us to the next point: Yes, a complete and balanced diet is essential to protect your and your baby's health. However, this should not degenerate into tense and insecure behavior. Putting every gram of meat or cheese on the gold scale will certainly not relax you. Over time, develop a feeling for a varied diet. The information and the delicious recipes in this book will help you here. And even if you have had a weak moment and resorted to fast food, the world will not end. Only as a rule it should definitely not become.

Tip 3: If you frequently find that you lack the desire to cook, you can of course also buy a small supply of food that you can prepare or defrost quickly and easily if necessary. This way you can quickly get a complete meal without having to force yourself to stand for hours at the stove in the kitchen.

Tip 4: Pay attention to your digestion. Do not put up with diarrhea, constipation or a permanent feeling of fullness. Be careful and ask yourself when the symptoms occur and which foods they may be associated with. Often heartburn & Co. can be prevented by minimal adjustments in your diet.

Tip 5: Take enough time for your meals. Especially if you are working, you should not take this point lightly. A quick trip to the canteen between two meetings is not a relaxing break. Consciously take the time for an undisturbed meal and chew every bite well. After all, in the end this is also good for your digestion and reduces the risk of digestive problems.

Tip 6: I cannot mention often enough how important a good nutritional balance is right now. You can best achieve this by buying regional and seasonal food. Long transport routes are eliminated, as is the frequent exposure to pesticides. Just find out if there is a farmer or farm store in your town or a neighboring town. Is there perhaps a weekly market that regularly offers regional products? I'm sure you will find what you're looking for if you make a targeted search.

Tip 7: Even if you can't find a farmer, make sure you buy organic products when you buy fruit and vegetables. They are demonstrably less contaminated with harmful substances and provide you and your baby with a higher proportion of nutrients and vital substances than fruit and vegetables without organic quality.

Tip 8: You may be familiar with the recommendation "five-a-day". This refers to five portions of fruit, salad or vegetables spread over the day, which you should eat. If you are unsure how large the amount should be, you can use your hand as a unit of measurement. 1 portion = 1 handful. This means you are on the safe side and can roughly estimate how much you should eat.

Tip 9: Prefer low-sodium, magnesium-rich mineral water, which is *not de-iced, as your* beverage. You can also drink still water if you suffer from heartburn.

Tip 10: Try to listen to your biorhythm. When does the body signal that it needs food (feeling hungry)? When do you feel fit and resilient? When do you need a break because the battery is empty? When do you get tired and need sleep?
Especially during pregnancy, be careful with your needs and do not simply ignore them. Your body is trying to tell you that it urgently needs something specific. For the sake of your well-being and that of your child, you should try to structure your daily routine according to your individual biorhythm. This alone is a valuable contribution to a more relaxed pregnancy.

Tip 11: If your pregnancy has gone without complications so far and you feel fit and balanced, there is nothing to stop you from going on a trip. The optimal time to travel is in the 2nd trimester, when the critical 1st trimester is over and the difficult 3rd trimester has not yet begun.

When choosing your vacation destination, however, be aware of possible risks of infection. Also, you should consider whether it must be now still absolutely a far journey or whether a vacation in the European foreign country does not bring also the desired recovery effect. A long journey time, jet lag and possible climate changes are no longer a problem. Beyond that also our beautiful Germany has quite attractive vacation goals, about which it is worth thinking.

Tip 12: Please consider that diarrhea is not uncommon abroad, especially due to a change in diet. Especially during pregnancy, you should of course take special care:

- Do not drink tap water; please also use the following for brushing your teeth Mineral water.
- It is best to avoid ice cubes completely; they often contain Pathogens.
- Especially in warm countries you drink enough mineral water, to avoid a lack of liquid.
- The consumption of perishable food, such as ice cream, mayonnaise or cream desserts you should also better postpone to home.
- It is best to peel fresh fruit.

"Peel it, fry it, boil it, or forget it!"

Basically, everything doesn't sound so difficult and quite feasible, does it?

Do`s & Don'ts in pregnancy - short & compact

Now you have almost completed the theoretical part of this guide. Finally, I would like to give you a short and concise overview of the most important "Do's and Don'ts". So, you have all the essential information at hand when you need to get started quickly. Let's start with the pleasant things, the Do's! You may now treat yourself to these, or you should pay special attention to them:

Do's:
- Hygiene in the kitchen
- Healthy nutrition
- rest and relaxation -> as often as possible
- Sex/ sexual intercourse (yes, this is also allowed!)
- Moderate sport/ exercise
- Exchange with other pregnant women (e.g. birth preparation course)
- pregnancy yoga, pelvic floor gymnastics, swimming course
- increased dental care

Don'ts:
- Alcohol and nicotine should be avoided during pregnancy and lactation strictly prohibited.
- Avoid stress and hectic.
- Do not practice any sports with increased risk of injury.
- For the duration of the pregnancy should not be dieting become.

- Consumption of white flour products and the consumption of sugar on a reduce minimum.
- Avoid ready salads from the bag, sprouts and seedlings as well as rotten vegetables and fruit.
- Reduce or completely avoid extremely fatty foods, fried foods, breaded foods, ready meals, fast food and sausages.
- Avoid raw meat, raw fish and raw milk products.
- "Food for 2" is not required.
- Avoid harsh/aggressive household cleaners and cleaning and disinfecting agents.

At this point in the book, you will have the necessary knowledge to turn your attention to the practical part of this guide.

So, let the many delicious recipes on the following pages encourage you to try them out and realize that in the end it is not so difficult to eat a balanced and healthy diet.

They now know which nutrients are hidden in which foods and can therefore ensure the targeted absorption of certain vitamins, trace elements and minerals.

Be patient with yourself and take your time to get used to the changed living conditions. After all, you now bear a great responsibility for your health and therefore inevitably also for that of your child.

Enjoy this very special time in your life and do something good for yourself as often as possible.

I hope that you were able to take a lot of interesting information from this book with you. I wish you a carefree pregnancy without complications and all the best for you and your baby.

Your Christine Rosenstein

P.S. I would be very happy about an evaluation of the book. Because it allows me to continue to live my dream of supporting young families successfully.

Recipes

Healthy and optimal nutrition during pregnancy

Drinks & Smoothies

Red Beet Juice

Servings: 2

Level of difficulty: easy

Ingredients

- 3 tubers beet
- 2 carrots
- 2 apples
- 1 piece of ginger (about 2 cm long)
- ½ Lemon

Preparation

1. Squeeze the lemon. Collect the juice with a sieve in a cup.
2. Peel the apples. Remove the core and the stem base and then grate the apples.
3. Peel and grate the carrots.
4. Peel and grate the ginger.
5. Peel and grate the beet. Make sure to put on kitchen gloves before doing so.
6. Put the rasps in a blender, add some water and mix everything. Press the finished mixture through a clean kitchen towel.
7. With a juicer it is enough to cut the ingredients into pieces. The machine does everything else.
8. Mix the juice with the lemon juice, pour into glasses and serve.

Beetroot Smoothie

Servings: 2

Level of difficulty: easy

Ingredients

- 4 beets
- 1 apple
- 1 piece of ginger (about 2 cm long)
- 200 ml apple juice
- 1 teaspoon cinnamon

Preparation

1. Peel the ginger and cut into small pieces.
2. Peel the apple. Remove the core and the stem base and then cut the apple into small pieces.
3. Peel the beet and cut into large cubes. Put them in a pot with 300 ml water and boil them for a quarter of an hour.
4. Remove the pot from the stove and let it cool down. Then put the beetroot with the water, the apple pieces, the ginger pieces, the apple juice and the cinnamon in a blender. Mix everything well. Pour the finished smoothie into matching glasses and serve.

Rhubarb-Strawberry Limo

Servings: 2

Level of difficulty: easy

Ingredients

- 3 sticks of rhubarb
- 100 g strawberries
- 3 leaves mint
- 1 tablespoon agave syrup

Preparation

1. Cut off about 1 cm of the rhubarb stalks at the end and beginning. Peel the sticks and cut them into about 2 cm small pieces.
2. Read out the strawberries. Remove the stalk base. Wash and quarter the strawberries.
3. Wash the mint and shake dry.
4. Put rhubarb pieces, strawberries, mint, the agave syrup and 50 ml water in a pot and let it simmer for 12 minutes.
5. Sift out the solid materials with a sieve. Collect the juice in a bowl.
6. Allow the juice to cool, mix with one liter of mineral water and then serve. Use the mint to garnish.

Lemon Ice Tea

Servings: 2

Level of difficulty: easy

Ingredients

- 1 lemon
- 1 sprig of lemon balm
- 2 leaves mint
- 1 tsp honey
- 2 bags of herbal tea

Preparation

1. Squeeze the lemon. Collect the juice with a sieve in a cup.
2. Wash the mint and lemon balm and shake dry.
3. Prepare the herbal tea with 1.5 liters of hot water. Leave to infuse for 10 minutes and then remove the tea bags.
4. Let the drink cool down.
5. Add the honey, lemon juice, mint and lemon balm. Leave the finished iced tea to steep in the refrigerator for one hour and then serve. On hot days, add ice cubes to the glasses.

Mint Ice Tea

Servings: 2

Level of difficulty: easy

Ingredients

- 4 sprigs of mint
- 1 tablespoon lemon juice
- 1 tsp honey

Preparation

1. Wash the mint and shake dry.
2. Bring 1 liter of water to the boil. Put the mint in a fireproof carafe, a pot or a pot. Pour the water over it. Add the lemon juice and honey. Stir briefly.
3. Allow the tea to cool to room temperature first and then place it in the refrigerator for an hour.
4. Serve the iced tea with ice cubes.

Blueberry Smoothie

Servings: 2

Level of difficulty: easy

Ingredients

- 150 g blueberries
- 1 apple
- 1 banana
- 100 g natural yoghurt

Preparation

1. Sort and wash the blueberries. Remove small remaining stems.
2. Peel the apple. Remove the core and the stem base and then cut the apple into narrow slices.
3. Peel the banana and cut into small pieces.
4. Put the blueberries, apple pieces and banana pieces in a blender. Add the yoghurt and 80 ml water. Mix everything well.
5. Pour the finished smoothie into matching glasses and serve.

Raspberry Lassi

Servings: 2

Level of difficulty: easy

Ingredients

- 100 g raspberries
- 125 g natural yogurt
- 50 ml milk
- 1 pinch of salt

Preparation

1. Select and wash the raspberries.
2. Put the raspberries in a blender. Add the yoghurt, milk and a pinch of salt. Mix everything well.
3. Pour the finished smoothie into matching glasses and serve.

Grapefruit-Kiwi Bowl

Servings: 2

Level of difficulty: easy

Ingredients

- 1 kiwi
- 1 grapefruit
- 1 tablespoon chia seeds
- 1 tsp honey

Preparation

1. Place the chia seeds in a bowl or small pot with 100 ml of water. Let them rest in the refrigerator for half an hour.
2. Peel the kiwi and cut into small pieces.
3. Cut the grapefruit in half and squeeze. Collect the juice with a sieve in a mixing cup.
4. Put the chia seed with the water in a mixing cup. Add the grapefruit juice, the kiwi pieces and the honey. Mix well and serve in glasses.

Watermelon-Lime Bowl

Servings: 2

Level of difficulty: easy

Ingredients

- 200 g watermelon (one large slice without skin or several small slices)
- ½ Lime
- 4 peppermint leaves
- 1 sprig of lemon balm
- 2 tablespoons cane sugar

Preparation

1. Cut the watermelon into small cubes.
2. Halve the lime and squeeze out one half.
3. Wash the peppermint and lemon balm and shake dry.
4. Mix 100 g of watermelon in a bowl with the lime juice, lemon balm and sugar. Let the mixture rest for one hour in a cool place.
5. Place the remaining 100 g watermelon in a blender jug. Add the peppermint and 50 ml mineral water. Mix the mixture well and put it in a cold place as well.
6. Mix both mixtures together, let it rest for an hour and then serve.

cherry lemonade

Servings: 2

Level of difficulty: easy

Ingredients

- 100 g fresh cherries
- 1 tablespoon agave syrup
- 1 tablespoon lemon juice
- 4 leaves mint

Preparation

1. Wash the mint and shake dry.
2. Wash the cherries. Remove the stalks and stone the cherries.
3. Put 1/3 of the cherries aside (approx. 30 g). Puree the other cherries with a blender. Mix the cherry puree with agave syrup, the lemon juice and 500 ml mineral water. Puree the mixture and place in the refrigerator for one hour.
4. Pour the cherry mixture into glasses. Divide the remaining cherries and mint into two glasses and serve.

Currant Cocktail

Servings: 2

Level of difficulty: easy

Ingredients

- 200 g currants
- 50 g raspberries
- 1 lime
- 2 sprigs of peppermint
- 1 tablespoon cane sugar
- 6 ice cubes

Preparation

1. Select and wash the currants and raspberries. If you use frozen goods, defrost them.
2. Cut open the lime and squeeze out the lime. Collect the juice.
3. Make crushed ice from 6 ice cubes with the mixer. Put the cane sugar, the currants and the raspberries into the blender jug with the crushed ice. Also add the peppermint and the lime juice. Mix everything well.
4. Put the juice in the refrigerator for one hour and then serve with ice cubes.

Yoghurt / Mango Lassi

Servings: 2

Level of difficulty: easy

Ingredients

- 150 g yoghurt (low-fat)
- 50 ml milk
- 1 tsp honey
- some cardamom
- 2 threads of saffron
- 100 ml mineral water
- 1 mango

Preparation

1. Put yoghurt, milk and honey in a blender. Add the cardamom, saffron and 100 ml mineral water. Mix everything well and serve fresh.
2. For a fruity mango lassi, puree a ripe mango and add to the other ingredients. You can also add a pinch of cinnamon to the mango lassi.

Summer Berry Shake

Servings: 2

Level of difficulty: easy

Ingredients

- 50 g strawberries
- 50 g raspberries
- 100 ml milk (low-fat)
- 2 tablespoons yoghurt (low-fat)
- 2 tablespoons honey

Preparation

1. Select and wash the strawberries and raspberries. If you use frozen goods, defrost them.
2. Put the berries in a blender. Add the milk, yogurt and honey. Mix everything well and serve fresh.

Berry Smoothie

Servings: 2

Level of difficulty: easy

Ingredients

- 1 orange
- 1 banana
- 100 g berry mixture (blueberries, raspberries or similar)
- 60 g beet
- 250 ml apple juice
- 250 ml mineral water

Preparation

1. Peel the beetroot and cut into small cubes.
2. Select and wash the berries. If you use frozen goods, defrost them.
3. Peel the orange and cut into small cubes. Remove the fibers.
4. Peel and slice the banana.
5. Put the beet with the berries, orange and banana in a blender. Add the apple juice and 250 ml mineral water. Mix the mixture thoroughly.
6. Pour the finished smoothie into matching glasses and serve.

Spinach-Mango-Smoothie

Servings: 2

Level of difficulty: easy

Ingredients

- 1 handful of leaf spinach
- 1 banana
- ½ Mango
- 250 ml orange juice
- 250 ml mineral water

Preparation

1. Wash, sort and chop the spinach.
2. Peel and slice the banana.
3. Peel the mango, remove the stone and cut half of the fruit into pieces. Keep the other half in the refrigerator.
4. Put the spinach with the banana pieces and the mango pieces in a blender. Add the orange juice and 250 ml mineral water. Mix everything well.
5. Pour the finished smoothie into matching glasses and serve.

Orange-Mango-Smoothie

Servings: 2

Level of difficulty: easy

Ingredients

- 2 oranges
- ½ Mango
- 1 carrot
- 1 tablespoon lemon juice
- 1 tsp honey
- 250 ml carrot juice
- 250 ml mineral water

Preparation

1. Peel the oranges and cut into small cubes. Remove the fibers.
2. Peel the carrot and cut into large pieces.
3. Peel the mango, remove the stone and cut half of the fruit into pieces. Keep the other half in the refrigerator.
4. Put the mango pieces, the orange and carrot pieces in a blender. Add the lemon juice, honey and carrot juice. Mix everything well.
5. Pour the finished smoothie into matching glasses and serve

Banana Salt Smoothie

Servings: 2

Level of difficulty: easy

Ingredients

- 1 handful lamb's lettuce
- 1 banana
- 1 apple
- 250 ml orange juice
- 250 ml mineral water

Preparation

1. Wash the salad, shake dry and chop into small pieces.
2. Peel and slice the banana.
3. Peel the apple. Remove the core and the stem base and then cut the apple into narrow slices.
4. Put the lamb's lettuce, apple and banana pieces in a blender. Add the orange juice and 250 ml mineral water. Mix everything well.
5. Pour the finished smoothie into matching glasses and serve.

Chia seed Smoothie

Servings: 2

Level of difficulty: easy

Ingredients

- 2 teaspoons chia seeds
- 1 orange
- 1 banana
- 1 handful of berries mixed (blueberries, raspberries etc.)
- 2 tablespoons yoghurt
- 5 g ginger
- 1 tablespoon oat flakes
- 250 ml almond milk

Preparation

1. Peel and slice the banana. Peel the orange and cut into small cubes. Remove the fibers. Sort and wash the berries. Defrost the frozen goods.
2. Peel and chop the ginger.
3. Put the chia seeds with the orange, banana pieces and yogurt in a blender. Add the ginger, the oat flakes and the almond milk. Mix everything well.
4. Pour the finished smoothie into matching glasses and serve.

Mango-Avocado-Smoothie

Servings: 2

Level of difficulty: easy

Ingredients

- 1 avocado
- ½ Mango
- 1 handful of spinach
- 250 ml almond milk

Preparation

1. Peel the mango, remove the stone and cut half of the fruit into pieces. Keep the other half in the refrigerator.
2. Cut the avocado in half, use a spoon to lift the inside out of both halves and put it into a mixing cup.
3. Put the mango pieces, spinach and almond milk into the blender jug. Mix everything well.
4. Pour the finished smoothie into matching glasses and serve.

Date Almond Smoothie

Servings: 2

Level of difficulty: easy

Ingredients

- 1 banana
- 4 dates
- 2 teaspoons baking cocoa
- 150 ml almond milk

Preparation

1. Cut the dates into small pieces.
2. Peel and slice the banana.
3. Put the banana pieces, the dates, the baking cocoa and the almond milk in a blender. Mix everything well.
4. Pour the finished smoothie into matching glasses and serve.

Elderberry Blossom Cocktail

Servings: 2

Level of difficulty: easy

Ingredients

- 5 leaves of lemon balm
- 1 lime
- 25 ml elderflower syrup
- 50 ml mineral water

Preparation

1. Wash the lemon balm and shake dry.
2. Squeeze the lime. Collect the juice with a sieve in a cup.
3. Pour the juice of the lime into a carafe. Add the elderflower syrup, lemon balm and mineral water.
4. Enjoy the mocktail fresh. On warm days add ice cubes.

Mango Margarita

Servings: 2

Level of difficulty: easy

Ingredients

- 6 raspberries
- 1 piece of ginger (approx. 2 cm long)
- 1 splash of lime juice
- 100 ml mango juice
- 100 ml grapefruit juice

Preparation

1. Peel and grate the ginger.
2. Select and wash the raspberries. Remove small remaining stems.
3. Put the raspberries with the grated ginger, lime juice, mango juice and grapefruit juice in a blender. Mix everything well.
4. Pour the finished juice into matching glasses and serve.

Blueberry Mojito non-alcoholic

Servings: 2

Level of difficulty: easy

Ingredients

- 125 g blueberries
- 3 limes
- 8 leaves fresh mint
- 2 teaspoons cane sugar
- 60 ml Ginger Ale
- 30 ml mineral water

Preparation

1. Select and wash the blueberries. Remove small remaining stems.
2. Squeeze the lime. Collect the juice with a sieve in a cup.
3. Wash the mint and shake dry.
4. Add the blueberries, lime juice, cane sugar, ginger ale and mineral water and mix well.
5. Pour the drink into a carafe. Add the mint.
6. Enjoy the non-alcoholic cocktail fresh. On warm days add ice cubes.

Ginger-Blood Orange Soda

Servings: 2

Level of difficulty: easy

Ingredients

- 3 blood oranges
- 1 piece of ginger (about 2 cm high)
- 2 tablespoons clover honey (or other honey)
- 500 ml mineral water

Preparation

1. Peel and grate the ginger.
2. Peel a blood orange and cut into narrow slices.
3. Halve 2 blood oranges and squeeze the juice. Use a sieve to sift out the seeds. Catch the juice in a bowl.
4. Pour the juice of the blood oranges, ginger, honey and mineral water into a carafe. Mix everything well.
5. Add the slices of blood orange to the drink.
6. Leave the drink in the refrigerator for two hours and serve.
7. Add ice cubes to the lemonade on hot days.

Strawberry freshness

Servings: 2

Level of difficulty: easy

Ingredients

- 150 g strawberries (fresh or sweet)
- 150 ml milk
- 3 tablespoons sweet cream
- 1 tsp maple syrup
- 1 teaspoon yeast flakes (high Vitamin B content)
- 1 pinch of cinnamon

Preparation

1. Sort and wash the strawberries. Remove the stalk. Cut the fruits into quarters. Use frozen food, defrost them first and then quarter them.
2. Put the strawberries, milk, yeast flakes and sweet cream in a blender and puree everything thoroughly. Pour the puree into a carafe.
3. Add the maple syrup and the cinnamon. Mix everything well.
4. Enjoy the fruity lemonade fresh.

Apricot Honey Drink

Servings: 2

Level of difficulty: easy

Ingredients

- 250 g apricots
- 2 teaspoons wildflower honey (or other honey)
- ½ l milk
- 200 ml mineral water

Preparation

1. Wash, halve and stone the apricots. Then puree the apricots in a mixer together with the mineral water.
2. Pour the apricot puree into a carafe. Add the milk and honey. Mix everything well.
3. Put the drink in the fridge for one hour and serve.

Orange Ice Shake

Servings: 2

Level of difficulty: easy

Ingredients

- 4 scoops of vanilla ice cream
- 40 ml chocolate syrup
- 20 ml orange syrup
- 250 ml milk
- Chocolate shavings

Preparation

1. Put the vanilla ice cream with the chocolate syrup, the orange syrup and the milk in a blender and mix well.
2. Serve the drink fresh and garnish with the chocolate shavings.

Three kinds of fruit lemonade

Servings: 2

Level of difficulty: easy

Ingredients

- 4 apples
- 4 pears
- 150 ml apple juice
- 150 ml cherry juice
- a pinch of cinnamon

Preparation

1. Peel the apples and the pears. Remove the core and the stem and then cut the fruit into small pieces.
2. Put the fruit in a mixer. Add the apple juice and cherry juice and puree well.
3. Serve the juice fresh. Garnish with a small pinch of cinnamon.

Limo on the Beach

Servings: 2

Level of difficulty: easy

Ingredients

- 200 ml pineapple juice
- 120 ml peach juice
- 60 ml cranberry syrup
- 6 ice cubes (from mineral water)

Preparation

1. Pour the pineapple juice with the peach juice and the cranberry syrup into a carafe. Mix all ingredients well.
2. Add the ice cubes and serve the drink.
3. Who likes can also make the juice from puree of fresh fruits. Add 250 - 300 ml of mineral water while pureeing.

Caipirinha non-alcoholic

Servings: 2

Level of difficulty: easy

Ingredients

- 2 organic limes
- 4 teaspoons cane sugar
- 80 ml Ginger Ale
- 120 ml passion fruit nectar
- freshly made crushed ice (from mineral water ice cubes)

Preparation

1. Wash the limes with hot water and then cut them into eighths.
2. Put the lime pieces into large caipirinha glasses. Add 2 teaspoons of cane sugar to each glass and fill the glass with crushed ice.
3. Mix the ginger ale with the passion fruit nectar and pour into the two glasses.
4. Serve the drink immediately. Add two large drinking straws.

Breakfast

Fried polenta slices

Servings: 2

Level of difficulty: easy

Ingredients

- Vegetable broth
- 125 g corn semolina
- Olive oil
- 1 garlic clove
- salt, pepper

Preparation

1. Prepare the vegetable stock with 500 ml hot water.
2. Peel and chop the garlic. In a large pot, add the vegetable broth and the garlic. Add heat and add the corn semolina to the boiling water. Stir all the time.
3. Season with salt and pepper. Cook the polenta for 45 minutes.
4. Brush a baking dish with oil. Fill the polenta dough into the dish and smooth it down.
5. Let the dough cool, take it out and put it on a kitchen board. Cut out round pieces of dough with baking tins.
6. Pour oil into a coated pan and heat. Fry the dough pieces for 6 minutes in the pan. Turn over after about 3 minutes.
7. Serve the finished polenta slices warm.

Exotic breakfast muesli

Servings: 2

Level of difficulty: easy

Ingredients

- 1 papaya
- 1 kiwi
- 1 persimmon
- 100 g coconut muesli
- 200 ml coconut water

Preparation

1. Peel the fruits and cut into large cubes.
2. Spread the muesli over two bowls. Add the coconut water and the fruit pieces. Mix everything well and serve immediately.

Goat cheese sandwich

Servings: 2

Level of difficulty: easy

Ingredients

- 4 goat gouda (made from heated milk!)
- 4 slices of whole grain toast
- 3 leaves frisée salad
- ½ Chicory
- 2 teaspoons Dijon mustard
- 1 tablespoon cranberries (glass)

Preparation

1. Wash the salad and shake dry.
2. Place two slices of whole grain toast on each plate. Spread the toast slices with the mustard.
3. Add some of the cranberries.
4. Then place the chicory and the frisée salad on top.
5. Finally, place the cheese on the slices of toast and serve.

Bruschetta with eggplants

Servings: 2

Level of difficulty: easy

Ingredients

- 2 eggplants
- 2 sprigs thyme
- 2 stems of basil
- 1 garlic clove
- 1 lemon
- 1 tablespoon of olive oil
- 4 slices of crusty bread

Preparation

1. Preheat the oven to 200 degrees (circulating air).
2. Cover a baking tray with baking paper.
3. Wash and halve the eggplants. Cut the flesh lengthwise with a sharp knife. Place the fruit halves on the baking paper.
4. Peel and chop the garlic. Squeeze the lemon. Wash the basil and thyme, shake dry and chop finely.
5. Apply the oil to the eggplant halves. Sprinkle the thyme, salt and pepper on the eggplants.
6. Cook the eggplants in the oven for three quarters of an hour.
7. Scrape out the flesh, chop finely, place in a bowl and sprinkle with lemon. Add the basil and garlic. Mix well and spread it on the bread. Serve like this.

Rolls with ricotta cream

Servings: 2

Level of difficulty: easy

Ingredients

- 125 g ricotta (made from pasteurized milk, packed from the supermarket)
- 1 bell pepper (yellow)
- 1 pickled gherkin
- 75 Turkey breast (smoked)
- 4 stems of basil
- ½ bunch of chives
- salt, pepper
- 2 wholemeal rye rolls

Preparation

1. Cut the rolls in half. If you like, you can bake them crispy in the oven for a few minutes before serving.
2. Drain the ricotta with a sieve.
3. Wash the peppers. Remove the stalk and core and then cut the peppers into narrow strips.
4. Wash the basil, shake dry and chop finely. Wash and chop the chives.
5. Cut the turkey breast into small cubes. Place them in a bowl. Dice paprika and gherkin and put them into the bowl. Add the herbs, salt and pepper. Mix everything well and spread on the rolls. Serve like this.

Muesli with wild rice

Servings: 2

Level of difficulty: easy

Ingredients

- 25 g wild rice
- 20 g apricots (dried)
- 5 tablespoons of Pauline barley
- 10 g oat flakes (firm)
- 3 tablespoons bulgur
- 20 cranberries (dried)
- 1 tsp maple syrup
- a pinch of salt
- Butter for the mould

Preparation

1. Preheat the oven to 200 degrees (circulating air).
2. Cut the apricots into small pieces.
3. Cook the wild rice in a pot of salted water for about 20 minutes. Then drain.
4. Spread a casserole dish with butter.
5. Put the apricots with the rice, the pearl barley and the oat flakes into the mold. Add the bulgur, the cranberries, the syrup, a pinch of salt and 1 liter of water. Mix everything well.
6. Cook the mixture in the oven for 90 minutes. Always stir once.
7. Take the muesli out of the oven and let it get cold. Then serve in a bowl with some milk.
8. The muesli can be kept for one week.

Fruit Quark Rolls

Servings: 2

Level of difficulty: easy

Ingredients

- 1 apple
- 1 lemon
- 10 tablespoons low-fat curd cheese
- 2 spring onions
- 2 tsp horseradish
- 2 teaspoons rape oil
- salt, pepper
- 2 rye rolls

Preparation

1. Cut the rolls in half. If you like, you can bake them crispy in the oven for a few minutes before serving.
2. Peel the apple. Remove the core and the stem base and then cut the apple into narrow slices.
3. Brown the apple slices on both sides in a pan greased with oil.
4. Wash the spring onions. Remove the roots and cut the onions into small rings.
5. Put the quark in a bowl. Add the horseradish.
6. Mix lemon, salt and pepper into the quark.
7. Place the apple slices on the bun halves. Pour the quark mixture on top and serve. If you like, you can also garnish the quark with fresh herbs.

Pine and Oat Crunchies

Servings: 2

Level of difficulty: easy

Ingredients

- 15 g pine nuts
- 50 g oat flakes (firm)
- 10 cherries, dried
- ¼ tsp cinnamon
- 10 ml honey
- 10 ml maple syrup
- ¼ tablespoon rapeseed oil
- a pinch of salt

Preparation

1. Preheat the oven to 200 degrees (circulating air).
2. Chop the pine nuts into small pieces. Alternatively, you can also use almonds.
3. Put the syrup, oil and honey in a pot and add so much heat until the mixture boils.
4. Mix oat flakes, cherries and pine nuts. Add the syrup-oil-honey stock to the mixture. Add a little salt.
5. Cover a baking tray with baking paper. Put the muesli mixture on top and put it in the oven for twenty minutes. Stir the mixture once every 3 to 5 minutes.
6. Take the muesli out of the oven and let it get cold. Then serve in a bowl with some milk. It can be kept for one week.

Egg Quark Wholemeal Roll

Servings: 2

Level of difficulty: easy

Ingredients

- 6 tablespoons low-fat curd cheese
- 4 salad leaves (depending on taste and offer)
- 1 lemon
- 4 tablespoons herbal mixture (Frankfurt herbs or similar)
- 2 eggs
- salt, pepper
- Paprika powder (noble sweet)
- 2 wholemeal rolls

Preparation

1. Hard boil the eggs, peel and slice them.
2. Squeeze the lemon. Collect the juice with a sieve in a cup.
3. Put the quark in a bowl. Add the herbs, lemon juice and eggs. Mix everything well.
4. Season with salt, paprika and pepper. Mix well once again.
6. Cut the rolls in half. If you like, you can bake them crispy in the oven for a few minutes before serving.
5. Place the salad on the bread roll halves. Put the curd mixture on top and serve.

Vanilla Nut Semolina

Servings: 2

Level of difficulty: easy

Ingredients

- 2 apples
- 50 g wholemeal wheat semolina
- 40 walnut kernels
- 1 tablespoon honey
- 1 teaspoon cinnamon
- 1 tablespoon cane sugar
- 1 vanilla pod

Preparation

1. Peel the apples. Remove the core and the stem base and then cut the apples into eight small pieces.
2. Put the apple pieces in a pot. Add honey, 4 tablespoons of water and the cinnamon. Bring to the boil briefly. Reduce the heat slightly and let everything steam for 6 minutes.
3. Scrape out the vanilla pod. Put the pulp aside.
4. Put the milk in a second pot. Add the vanilla pulp and some salt. Mix well and bring the mixture to the boil briefly.
5. Mix the semolina with the sugar and add it to the hot milk. Whisk with an egg whisk.
6. Chop the walnut kernels into small pieces and add to the semolina. Add the apple pieces. Mix everything well and serve.

Chicken Salad

Servings: 2

Level of difficulty: easy

Ingredients

- 1 slice of pineapple (tin)
- 2 onions (red)
- 12 mushrooms
- 200 g chicken breast (smoked, cold cuts)
- 300 g yoghurt
- 4 stems tarragon
- 100 g alfalfa sprouts
- 2 wholemeal baguette rolls

Preparation

1. Peel and chop the onion.
2. Clean the mushrooms and dice them as well.
3. Cut the pineapple slice into small cubes.
4. Wash the tarragon, shake dry and chop finely.
5. Put the mushrooms, pineapple pieces, mushrooms and chicken breast in a bowl. Add the yoghurt, herbs and onions. Season with salt and pepper. Mix everything well.
6. Sort the sprouts, wash and shake dry.
7. Cut the rolls in half. If you like, you can bake them crispy in the oven for a few minutes before serving.
8. First place the sprouts on the bun halves and then apply the mushroom-chicken mixture with a spoon. Serve like this.

Avocado cream cheese spread

Servings: 2

Level of difficulty: easy

Ingredients

- 1 avocado
- 2 carrots
- 2 lemons
- 2 tablespoons cream cheese
- 2 small cucumbers
- salt, pepper
- 4 slices of wholemeal spelt bread

Preparation

1. Cut the avocado in half, use a spoon to lift out the inside and put it in a small bowl. Squeeze the lemon. Collect the juice in a cup with a sieve and pour it onto the avocado.
2. Peel the carrots and grate them with a vegetable grater.
3. Place the avocado in a bowl with the carrot shavings. Add the cream cheese. Season with salt and pepper. Mix everything well.
4. Peel the cucumbers and cut them into thin slices.
5. Place the cucumber slices on the bread. Pile up the cream cheese mixture on top. Garnish with fresh herbs and serve.

Chickpea Pancakes

Servings: 2

Level of difficulty: easy

Ingredients

- 300 g chickpeas flour
- 5 OIL
- Oil for frying
- 500 ml soy milk
- 1 teaspoon salt
- a pinch of sugar

Preparation

1. Mix the soy milk with the chickpea flour.
2. Add 5 tablespoons of oil, the salt and some sugar to the dough. Mix everything well.
3. Put oil in a pan, heat it up and use a ladle to pour the dough into the hot pan. Bake the pancakes until golden brown. Turn the pancakes over with a spatula and bake from the other side.
4. Place the finished pancakes on a plate and serve while still warm.
5. Spread with cinnamon, sugar, maple syrup, apple sauce or fruit jam, depending on taste.

Hazelnut Puree

Servings: 2

Level of difficulty: easy

Ingredients

- 250 g hazelnuts
- a pinch of cinnamon
- 6 dried dates
- 2 tablespoons maple syrup

Preparation

1. Preheat the oven to 200 degrees (circulating air).
2. Cover a baking tray with baking paper.
3. Put the hazelnuts on the baking paper and put them in the oven for twenty minutes.
4. Cut the dates into small pieces.
5. Let the nuts cool down.
6. Remove the shell from the nuts. It should now come off very easily. Put the nuts in a blender and chop them up.
7. Put the nut flour in a bowl and mix it with the cinnamon, dates and maple syrup. Mix everything well once again.
8. Pour the finished nutmeg into previously hot rinsed disposable glasses. Place this on the breakfast table and enjoy it.

Wheat bran with fruit mixture

Servings: 2

Level of difficulty: easy

Ingredients

- 100 g oat flakes
- 200 ml oat milk
- 1 banana
- ½ TL Vanilla pulp (freshly scraped out of a vanilla pod or vanilla extract)
- 4 tablespoons wheat bran
- 3 teaspoons maple syrup

Preparation

1. Peel the banana and cut it into small pieces.
2. Put the oat flakes in a pot. Add the goat milk, vanilla extract and 150 ml water. Mix everything well and bring the mixture to the boil.
3. Reduce the heat and simmer the porridge for ten minutes. Always stir.
4. Take the porridge from the stove and let it cool down.
5. Fill the porridge in two bowls. Add the banana pieces, wheat bran and maple syrup and serve the porridge as it is. You can add more pieces of fruit if you wish.

Mango Bowl

Servings: 2

Level of difficulty: easy

Ingredients

- 1 banana
- ½ Mango
- ½ avocado
- 2 tablespoons oat flakes

Preparation

1. Put the oat flakes in a small bowl. Add some water and soak the oat flakes for 10 minutes.
2. Peel and slice the banana.
3. Peel the mango, remove the stone and cut half of the fruit into pieces. Keep the other half in the refrigerator.
4. Cut the avocado in half, use a spoon to lift the inside out of one half and put it into a mixing cup. Keep the other half in the refrigerator.
5. Put half of the banana slices and the avocado pieces into the blender jug. Puree everything well. Add some mineral water if necessary.
6. Put the fruit puree in bowls and put the oat flakes on top. Decorate the bowl with the banana slices.

Fruit Porridge

Servings: 2

Level of difficulty: easy

Ingredients

- 250 g mixed berries (depending on season and offer, fresh or sweet)
- 250 ml milk
- 1 apple
- 1 handful of nuts
- 2 tsp raisins
- 2 teaspoons linseed
- 100 g oat flakes (or also millet flakes)

Preparation

1. Select and wash the berries. Remove small remaining stalks. Defrost the frozen goods.
2. Peel the apple. Remove the core and the stem base and then cut the apple into small pieces.
3. Pour the milk into a pot. Add the apple pieces, the nuts, the raisins and the linseed. Heat the mixture and simmer for a few minutes.
4. Add the oat flakes to the mixture. Stir well. Simmer for three minutes.
5. Remove the porridge from the stove and let it cool down.
6. Fill the porridge into bowls. Sprinkle the berries over it and serve.

Iron Power Breakfast

Servings: 2

Level of difficulty: easy

Ingredients

- 200 g soy yoghurt
- 30 g amaranth (contains protein, unsaturated fatty acids, important minerals)
- 1 tablespoon linseed
- 1 tablespoon linseed oil
- 1El agave syrup
- 1 teaspoon Acai powder
- 1 teaspoon baobab powder
- 4 pecan nuts
- 1 banana
- 3 tablespoons blueberries
- 1 tablespoon coconut flakes

Preparation

1. Sort and wash the blueberries. Remove small remaining stems. Peel and slice the banana. Chop the nuts into small pieces.
2. Mix the yogurt in a bowl with the amaranth, linseed oil, agave syrup, acai and babobab powder.
3. In two glasses alternately layer the yoghurt mixture and the fruit.
4. Roast the coconut flakes in a pan without fat and then put them on top of the layers in the glasses. Serve like this.

Breakfast rolls

Servings: 2

Level of difficulty: easy

Ingredients

- 400 g low-fat curd cheese
- 4 eggs
- 100 g oatmeal
- 80 g wheat bran
- 140 g spelt flour
- 2 tsp salt
- 4 teaspoons baking powder
- 40 g flea seed husks

Preparation

1. Preheat the oven to 175 degrees (circulating air).
2. Place the low-fat curd cheese in a bowl. Beat the eggs and add them. Also add the oat bran, wheat bran, spelt flour, psyllium husks, salt and baking powder to the bowl.
3. Heat 180 ml water and add to the mixture. Knead everything well.
4. Cover the dough with a kitchen towel and leave to rise for an hour in a warm place.
5. Form rolls from the dough and bake them in the oven. The baking time is about 45 minutes.
6. Serve the rolls still warm.

Oat flakes with fruit and nuts

Servings: 2

Level of difficulty: easy

Ingredients

- 50 g oat flakes
- 150 g natural yoghurt
- 200 g strawberries
- ½ Mango & ½ Orange
- 10 g linseed
- 150 g cashew nuts
- 2 tsp honey

Preparation

1. Peel and halve the orange and cut it into small cubes. Keep one half in the refrigerator.
2. Peel the mango, remove the stone and cut half of the fruit into pieces. Keep the other half in the refrigerator.
3. Sort and wash the strawberries. Remove the stalk attachments. Cut the fruits into quarters.
4. Put 100 g cashew nuts into a blender. Add 50 ml mineral water. Puree the nuts.
5. Put 25 g oatmeal in a bowl with a little water. Add the yoghurt, honey and nutmeg. Mix everything well and distribute in two bowls.
6. Add orange pieces, strawberries and mango pieces to the muesli. Place the bowls in the refrigerator overnight and serve early for breakfast. Sprinkle the remaining oatmeal and flax seed on top.

Appetizers

Bruschetta

Servings: 2

Level of difficulty: easy

Ingredients

- 2 ½ Meat tomatoes
- 1 ciabatta bread
- 1 garlic clove
- 1 ½ tablespoon of olive oil
- Salt
- Pepper

Preparation

1. Preheat the oven to 200 degrees (circulating air).
2. Wash the tomatoes. Remove the stalk and then cut the tomatoes into small pieces. Peel and chop the garlic.
3. Mix pepper and salt with ½ tsp olive oil. You need about ¼ teaspoon salt and as much pepper. Freshly ground pepper is best.
4. Put the tomatoes in a bowl. Mix in the spice mixture and garlic. Place the tomato pieces in the refrigerator for 2 hours.
5. Cover a baking tray with baking paper.
6. Cut the ciabatta into thick slices. Sprinkle the remaining oil on these slices.
7. Spoon the tomato pieces onto the ciabatta pieces. Put them in the oven for 10 minutes.
8. Take them out of the oven and place them on a large plate. Decorate the slices with fresh herbs.

Rocket Wrap

Servings: 2

Level of difficulty: easy

Ingredients

- 2 tortillas
- 2 handfuls of rocket
- 1 large carrot
- 6 tablespoons of ricotta (made from pasteurized milk, packed from the supermarket)
- salt, pepper

Preparation

1. Sort the rocket, wash and shake dry.
2. Peel the carrot and grate it with a vegetable grater.
3. Put the rocket on baking paper and cover with rocket. Put the grated carrots on top.
4. Apply the ricotta to the grated carrots. Sprinkle with salt and pepper.
5. Roll up the tortilla without baking paper and put it on a plate. Serve it like this.

Spinach cream soup

Servings: 2

Level of difficulty: easy

Ingredients

- 100 g peas (tin or tin)
- 100 g spinach
- 15 g butter
- some flour
- ¼ tablespoon rapeseed oil
- 60 ml cream
- 250 ml beef broth
- salt, pepper

Preparation

1. Frozen Defrost peas. Use canned peas, drain them and rinse briefly.
2. Wash, sort and chop the spinach.
3. Prepare the broth.
4. Melt the butter in a pan. Add the flour and mix. Do not add too much heat. Deglaze with the broth. Let everything simmer for about 5 minutes.
5. Add the spinach. Simmer for 10 minutes and then add the peas. Let everything simmer for another 10 minutes. Season with salt and pepper.
6. Puree the soup with a hand blender. Season to taste and add seasoning if necessary. Serve on a deep plate. Garnish with a spoon of cream.

Chickpea salad

Servings: 2

Level of difficulty: easy

Ingredients

- 200 g chick peas
- ½ Cucumber
- ½ Bunch of spring onions
- 2 carrots
- 1 paprika
- 2 tablespoons lemon juice
- salt, pepper

Preparation

1. Drain the chickpeas and rinse briefly.
2. Peel and halve the cucumber. Cut one half into small slices.
3. Wash the spring onions. Remove the roots and cut the onions into small rings.
4. Peel the carrots and cut into small rings.
5. Wash the peppers. Remove the stalk and core and then cut the peppers into narrow strips.
6. Place the vegetables in a large bowl. Add the lemon juice. Season with salt and pepper. Stir well.
7. Season to taste and if necessary, add salt and pepper.
8. Leave the salad to stand in the refrigerator for an hour and then serve. Sprinkle a few croutons over the salad.

Vanilla Quark

Servings: 2

Level of difficulty: easy

Ingredients

- 200 g quark (20% fat content)
- 150 g natural yoghurt (3.5% fat content)
- 1 apple
- 50 g millet flakes
- 1 package vanilla sugar
- 1 tsp lemon juice
- 2 tablespoons raisins

Preparation

1. Peel the apple and grate it with a vegetable grater. Put the grated apples in a bowl.
2. Add the quark and yoghurt to the apple and mix well. Add the vanilla sugar, lemon juice and raisins and mix well once again.
3. Serve the quark in small bowls. Sprinkle the small bowls with the millet flakes.

Beet salad

Servings: 2

Level of difficulty: easy

Ingredients

- 400 g beet
- 1 orange
- 20 g walnut kernels
- 2 tablespoons walnut oil
- 2 tablespoons orange juice
- 1 teaspoon creamed horseradish
- 2 slices of wholemeal bread
- salt, pepper (freshly ground)

Preparation

1. Peel the beetroot and cut into small cubes. Put them into a bowl.
2. Peel the orange and cut into small cubes. Remove the fibers and add the orange pieces to the beetroot.
3. Add the walnut oil and orange juice to the bowl. Also add the horseradish. Mix everything together well. Season with salt and pepper.
4. Mix in the walnuts. Let the salad stand for an hour and season to taste.
5. Put the slices of wholemeal bread on small plates and place the salad on top. Serve like this.

Raw vegetable salad

Servings: 2

Level of difficulty: easy

Ingredients

- 150 g rocket salad
- 1 paprika
- 1 carrot
- 250 g cocktail tomatoes
- 20 g sprouts mix

Preparation

1. Sort the rocket, wash and shake dry.
2. Wash the peppers. Remove the stalk and core and then cut the peppers into narrow strips.
3. Peel the carrot and cut into small rings.
4. Wash and quarter the cocktail tomatoes.
5. Sort out the sprout mix, rinse, shake dry and place in a large bowl. Add the vegetables. Mix everything well and then divide into two plates.
6. Garnish with a light dressing, some yogurt or a few herbs, depending on your mood.

Cream Cheese Cress Balls

Servings: 2

Level of difficulty: easy

Ingredients

- 1 box cress
- 100 g heavy cream cheese
- 1 tablespoon sesame seed
- 1 pinch of salt

Preparation

1. Cut off the cress, wash and shake dry.
2. Sprinkle the cress onto a plate. Sprinkle the sesame seeds and salt over it.
3. Roll small balls out of the cheese and roll them over the cress-sesame mixture.
4. Spread the cream cheese cress balls on a plate and serve.

Millet Cookies

Servings: 2

Level of difficulty: easy

Ingredients

- 100 g millet
- ½ bunch of parsley
- 1 egg (organic)
- 3 tablespoons oat flakes
- 2 tablespoons sesame seed
- 1 tablespoon of olive oil
- a little paprika powder (sweet)
- salt, pepper

Preparation

1. Wash the parsley, shake dry and chop finely.
2. Simmer the millet in a pot of salted water for about 20 minutes until it is cooked. Then drain and let it cool down a little.
3. Place the millet in a bowl. Add the egg, the oatmeal, the sesame and the parsley. Add the oil as well. Mix everything well. Season with salt, paprika and pepper. Season to taste and add more if necessary.
4. Let the salad steep a little and then serve on plates or in salad bowls.

Basil mozzarella balls

Servings: 2

Level of difficulty: easy

Ingredients

- 4 dried tomatoes
- 5 sprigs of basil
- 100 g mozzarella balls
- 1 tablespoon of olive oil
- 1 tablespoon of Aceto Balsamic
- salt, pepper

Preparation

1. Wash the basil, shake dry and chop finely.
2. Dice the tomatoes and put them in a bowl. Add the basil, oil and vinegar. Add the mozzarella balls. Season with salt and pepper.
3. Season to taste and add seasoning if necessary. Put the balls on a plate with the tomato-basil mixture and serve.

Tomato and lentil soup

Servings: 2

Level of difficulty: easy

Ingredients

- 1 stick of leek
- 100 g red lentils
- 100 g cocktail tomatoes
- Vegetable broth
- 200 g chopped tomatoes (tin)
- 4 sprigs of basil
- Cayenne pepper
- 3 tablespoons sour cream
- salt, pepper

Preparation

1. Wash the leeks. Remove the roots and cut the onions into small rings.
2. Wash and quarter the cocktail tomatoes.
3. Wash the basil, shake dry and chop finely.
4. Prepare the vegetable stock with 250 ml hot water.
5. Put the oil in a pot and fry the leeks in it. Deglaze with the vegetable broth.
6. Add the chopped tomatoes, cocktail tomatoes and lentils to the pot and simmer for a quarter of an hour. Season with salt, cayenne pepper and pepper.
7. Season to taste and if necessary, add salt and pepper. Serve the soup on deep plates and garnish with basil and some sour cream.

Paprika beef strips

Servings: 2

Level of difficulty: easy

Ingredients

- 250 g beef rump steak
- 1 small onion
- 1 red bell pepper
- 2 tablespoons olive oil
- ¼ teaspoon paprika powder (sweet)
- some branches of rosemary
- some branches of thyme
- salt, pepper

Preparation

1. Peel the onion and cut into small cubes.
2. Wash the peppers. Remove the stalk and core and then cut into narrow strips.
3. Wash the rosemary and thyme, shake dry and chop finely.
4. Cut the beef rump steak with a sharp knife into very fine strips.
5. In a bowl, mix 1 tablespoon of oil with paprika and the herbs, put the meat in it and let it rest for half an hour.
6. Heat the remaining oil in a frying pan. Sauté the paprika and onion in it. Season with salt and pepper. Add the strips of meat and fry well.
7. Remove the meat strips, put them into small bowls and serve. Serve with soup and some fresh salad.

Marinated chicken skewers

Servings: 2

Level of difficulty: easy

Ingredients

- 300 g chicken breast fillets
- ¼ TL coriander seed
- ¼ TL peppercorns
- red pepper berries
- 2 tablespoons olive oil
- 1 tsp lime juice
- Salt
- 4 wooden skewers

Preparation

1. Rinse the chicken breast fillet, dab dry with kitchen paper and cut lengthwise into 6 - 8 long strips.
2. Chop the peppercorns, pepper berries and coriander into a mortar. Mix the spice mixture in a small bowl with oil and lime juice and spread it on the chicken strips. Leave the meat to soak in a cool place for half an hour.
3. Place the meat on the skewers in a wave shape and fry in a pan with hot oil. Season with salt.
4. Serve the skewers with a fresh salad.

Beet egg salad

Servings: 2

Level of difficulty: easy

Ingredients

- 2 beet
- 1 avocado
- 4 eggs
- 1 bunch of chives
- 2 tablespoons flaked almonds
- 2 tablespoons balsamic vinegar
- 1 tablespoon of olive oil
- 6 tablespoons buttermilk
- 1 tablespoon mayonnaise
- salt, pepper, cayenne pepper

Preparation

1. In a small bowl, mix the balsamic vinegar with the olive oil, buttermilk, mayonnaise and a little salt, pepper and cayenne pepper.
2. Boil the eggs hard, quench, peel and slice them.
3. Peel the avocado. Remove the core. Cut the fruit into pieces.
4. Wash and chop the chives.
5. Roast the flaked almonds in a pan without fat.
6. Place the beet on two plates. Place the eggs and the avocado on top. Sprinkle with the chives and the flaked almonds.
7. Pour the dressing over it

Kohlrabi soup

Servings: 2

Level of difficulty: easy

Ingredients

- 1 kohlrabi
- 1 onion
- 400 g potatoes
- Vegetable broth
- 100 ml cream
- ½ bunch of parsley
- Nutmeg
- salt, pepper

Preparation

1. Prepare the vegetable stock with 500 ml hot water.
2. Wash the parsley, shake dry and chop finely.
3. Peel and chop the kohlrabi and the potatoes. Peel and chop the onion.
4. Sauté the onion in a pan with hot oil until it is golden yellow. Add the kohlrabi and potato pieces and fry well. Deglaze with the vegetable stock. Let everything simmer for 25 minutes. Season with salt and pepper and puree with a blender.
5. Add the parsley and the cream. Mix everything well. Add a little nutmeg. Season to taste and if necessary, add salt and pepper.
6. Serve the soup on deep plates.

Marinated zucchinis

Servings: 2

Level of difficulty: easy

Ingredients

- 750 g zucchini
- 3 stems of mint
- ½ Lemon
- 2 tablespoons honey
- 2 tablespoons olive oil
- salt, pepper

Preparation

1. Wash the mint, shake dry and chop finely.
2. Peel and slice the zucchini.
3. Squeeze the lemon. Collect the juice with a sieve in a cup.
4. Add 1 tablespoon of oil, honey and mint to the lemon juice. Mix everything well.
5. Put the remaining oil in a pan and lightly brown the zucchini slices on both sides.
6. Spread the marinade on the zucchini slices and fry the zucchini slices again.
7. Place the finished zucchini slices on two plates and serve.

Marinated olives

Servings: 2

Level of difficulty: easy

Ingredients

- 350 g olives (green)
- 200 g fennel
- 1 onion (red)
- 1 chili pepper
- 1 orange
- ½ Basil bunch
- 2 tablespoons olive oil
- Pepper

Preparation

1. Cut the olives with a knife and put them in a bowl.
2. Remove the stalk of the chili pepper. Cut the chili pepper open lengthwise, remove the seeds and then chop the pepper into small pieces.
3. Peel the onion and cut into small rings.
4. Wash and clean the fennel. Remove the stalk and cut the fennel into small cubes.
5. Wash the basil, shake dry and chop finely.
6. Peel the orange, cut it in half and squeeze the juice.
7. Add onions, chili and fennel to the olives. Add the orange juice, oil, a little pepper and basil. Mix everything well and let it stand in the refrigerator for 2 days. Then put them in small bowls and serve.

Asparagus raw food

Servings: 2
Level of difficulty: easy

Ingredients

- 100 g potatoes (firm boiling)
- ½ Lemon
- ½ avocado
- 200 g asparagus (white and green)
- 80 g purslane
- 1 tablespoon tahini
- 100 g yoghurt (1.5 % fat content)

Preparation

1. Peel potatoes, cut into small cubes and cook in salted water until al dente. Then drain the water and put the potatoes in a large bowl.
2. Cut the avocado in half, use a spoon to lift out the inside and put it in a small bowl. Squeeze the lemon. Collect the juice in a cup with a sieve and pour it onto the avocado.
3. Wash, clean and shake dry the purslane.
4. Peel the asparagus, cut off the end and then cut the asparagus into small pieces about 1 - 2 cm long.
5. Add the asparagus, purslane and avocado pieces to the potatoes in the bowl.
6. Add the tahin, yogurt, remaining lemon juice, salt and pepper. Mix everything together well. Leave the salad to stand in a cool place for an hour and then serve.

Asparagus-Tomato Salad

Servings: 2

Level of difficulty: easy

Ingredients

- 500 g asparagus (white)
- 200 g cherry tomatoes
- 1 lemon
- 1 bunch of dill
- 2 tablespoons olive oil
- 1 teaspoon agave syrup
- salt, pepper

Preparation

1. Squeeze the lemon. Collect the juice with a sieve in a cup.
2. Wash the tomatoes and cut them into small pieces.
5. Wash the dill, shake dry and chop into small pieces.
3. Peel the asparagus, cut off the end and then cut the asparagus into small pieces about 1 - 2 cm long.
4. Cook the asparagus pieces in a pot of salted water for 6 minutes until they are firm to the bite. Then drain the water and put the asparagus in a large bowl.
5. Add the tomatoes and the dill. Also add the lemon juice, olive oil and agave syrup. Season with salt and pepper. Mix everything well.
6. Leave to stand for a few minutes and then serve.

Pear-Endive Salad

Servings: 2

Level of difficulty: easy

Ingredients

- 150 g endive salad
- 1 bulb
- 4 tablespoons pear juice
- 1 tablespoon rapeseed oil
- 2 tablespoons cream cheese
- 40 g walnuts
- salt, pepper

Preparation

1. Sort the endive salad, wash and shake dry.
2. Peel and chop the pear.
3. Roast the walnuts in a pan without fat.
4. Put the endive salad in a large bowl. Add the pear pieces and the cream cheese. Mix everything well.
5. In a cup or small bowl, mix the rape seed oil with the pear juice. Add salt and pepper. Mix well and pour the dressing into the bowl. Once again mix everything well, leave to stand for half an hour and then serve.

Main courses for lunch and dinner

Plaice with spinach

Servings: 2

Level of difficulty: easy

Ingredients

- 150 g leaf spinach
- 3 stems dill
- 360 g plaice fillet
- 1 onion
- 1 lemon
- 75 g prawns (North Sea or according to offer)
- 1 tablespoon of oil
- salt, pepper

Preparation

1. Wash the dill, shake dry and chop into small pieces. Wash, sort and chop the spinach. Rinse the fish fillet, dab dry with kitchen paper and salt and pepper on both sides.
2. Fry the plaice fillet in a pan with hot oil on both sides.
3. Remove the fillet from the pan and put it aside.
4. Peel and chop the onion. Sauté the onion in a pan with hot oil. Add the spinach to the pan and fry for three minutes. Add salt, pepper and lemon to the spinach. Stir well and season to taste.
5. Rinse the shrimps and fry them in a pan with hot oil. Then mix into the spinach.
6. Serve the crab spinach with the fish fillet. Serve with a baked baguette and a fresh salad.

Pasta with salmon and asparagus vegetables

Servings: 2

Level of difficulty: easy

Ingredients

- 250 g ribbon noodles (whole grain)
- 300 g asparagus
- 1 onion
- 2 salmon fillets (approx. 125 g)
- Vegetable broth
- 100 g cream cheese
- 1 tsp lemon juice
- salt, pepper

Preparation

1. Prepare the vegetable stock with 150 ml hot water. Peel and chop the onion.
2. Peel the asparagus, cut off the ends and then cut the asparagus into small pieces about 1 - 2 cm long.
3. Rinse the fish fillet, dab dry with kitchen paper and salt and pepper on both sides.
4. Fry the onion and garlic in a pan with hot oil.
5. Cook the noodles in salted water for about 10 minutes until they are al dente, then drain.
6. Add the asparagus to the pan and steam for 5 minutes. Add the fish, steam briefly (about 2 minutes) and deglaze with the vegetable stock.
7. Let the fish and asparagus pan simmer for another 5 minutes. Before that, add the cream cheese, salt, pepper and lemon juice.
8. Pour the pasta into the pan, toss and serve.

Spätzle with steak

Servings: 2
Level of difficulty: easy

Ingredients

- 200 g wholemeal spaetzle
- 300 g minced pork steak
- 1 onion
- 2 peppers (yellow and red)
- 1 tablespoon of olive oil
- Vegetable broth
- 100 ml strained tomatoes
- 3 sprigs each of thyme and rosemary
- 2 tablespoons sour cream
- salt, pepper, paprika powder (rose hot)

Preparation

1. Peel and chop the onion. Wash the peppers. Remove the stalk and core and then cut the peppers into narrow strips. Prepare the vegetable stock with 150 ml hot water.
2. Wash the herbs, shake them dry and chop them finely.
3. Fry the steaks briefly and thoroughly in a pan with hot oil. Then remove the meat from the pan and keep warm in the preheated oven.
4. Sauté the onion in the pan. Add some oil if necessary. Add the peppers to the pan and fry for 5 minutes. Season with salt and pepper.
5. Place the meat in the pan. Add the tomatoes, cream and vegetable stock to the pan. Add paprika, rosemary and thyme. Steam everything for 5 minutes, lick off, season if necessary and then serve.

Tuna Steaks

Servings: 2

Level of difficulty: easy

Ingredients

- 250 g tuna steaks
- 2 leeks
- ½ Lemon
- 50 g crème fraiche
- 2 tablespoons butter
- 50 ml water
- salt, pepper
- Baguette

Preparation

1. Wash the leeks. Remove the roots and cut the onions into small rings.
2. Rinse the tuna fillet, dab dry with kitchen paper and salt and pepper on both sides.
3. Halve the lemon and squeeze one half. Collect the juice with a sieve in a cup. Keep the second half of the lemon in the refrigerator.
4. Sauté the leek in a pan with hot butter. Deglaze with 50 ml water. Add crème fraiche, salt and pepper and simmer covered for 10 minutes.
5. Add the steaks to the vegetables, cook for 15 minutes at reduced heat and then serve.
6. Serve with couscous or a baguette baked in the oven.

Goulash Hungarian

Servings: 2

Level of difficulty: easy

Ingredients

- 250 g pork goulash
- 2 onions
- 1 garlic clove
- 1 paprika
- Vegetable broth
- ½ Cup of sour cream
- 25 g margarine
- 1 tablespoon tomato paste
- salt, pepper, paprika powder (sweet)

Preparation

1. Preheat the oven to 200 degrees (circulating air).
2. Peel and chop the onions. Wash the peppers. Peel and chop the garlic. Remove the stalk and core and then cut the peppers into narrow strips. Prepare the vegetable stock with 150 ml hot water.
3. Fry the onion and garlic in a pan with margarine. Sauté the meat. Add the paprika and tomato paste. Season with salt, paprika powder and pepper.
4. Deglaze with the vegetable stock. Put the vegetables together with the meat and liquid in a Roman casserole dish and place in the oven for 90 minutes.

Salmon with coconut-vegetable puree

Servings: 2

Level of difficulty: easy

Ingredients

- 2 salmon fillets (approx. 300 g)
- 300 g potatoes (floury cooking)
- 200 g parsnips
- 200 ml coconut milk
- salt, pepper

Preparation

1. Peel the parsnips and cut into small cubes.
2. Peel the potatoes, cut them into small cubes and cook them together with the parsnips in salted water until al dente. Then drain the water and mash the parsnips and potatoes with a potato masher. Season with salt and pepper. Add 100 ml coconut milk. Stir well. Season to taste, if necessary, season with salt and pepper.
3. Rinse the fish fillet, dab dry with kitchen paper and salt and pepper on both sides.
4. Put half of the coconut milk in a pan, add heat and cook the fish in the pan.
5. Serve the puree with the fish.

Paprika pan

Servings: 2

Level of difficulty: easy

Ingredients

- 2 peppers
- ½ Onion
- 1 carrot
- 200 g minced meat (mixed)
- 1 tablespoon tomato paste
- ½ bunch of parsley
- 2 tablespoons sour cream

Preparation

1. Peel and chop the onion. Wash the peppers. Remove the stalk and core and then cut the peppers into narrow strips. Peel the carrots and cut them into small rings.
2. Wash the parsley, shake dry and chop finely.
3. Sauté the onion in a pan with hot oil. Add the minced meat. Season with salt and pepper.
4. Add the vegetables to the pan and fry for 6 minutes. Mix everything well. Deglaze with 100 ml water.
5. Put the paprika-meat mixture on two plates. Garnish with sour cream and parsley.

Spaghetti with salmon

Servings: 2

Level of difficulty: easy

Ingredients

- 125 g salmon fillet
- 250 g spaghetti
- 1 zucchini
- ½ Lemon
- ½ tablespoons olive oil
- salt, pepper

Preparation

1. Rinse the fish fillet, dab dry with kitchen paper and salt and pepper on both sides.
2. Peel and slice the zucchini.
3. Cut the lemon into slices.
4. Fry the zucchini strips in a pan with hot oil. After a few minutes add the salmon. Season with salt and pepper.
5. Cook the pasta in salted water until al dente, drain and serve. Serve with the fish. Garnish the plates with the lemon slices.

Potato soup with sausages

Servings: 2

Level of difficulty: easy

Ingredients

- 750 g potatoes (floury cooking)
- ½ Onion
- 1 small carrot
- 4 Vienna sausages
- ¼ bunch parsley
- Vegetable broth
- Sunflower oil
- salt, pepper, marjoram

Preparation

1. Peel potatoes and cut into small cubes. Peel and chop the onion. Peel the carrots and cut into small rings. Wash the parsley, shake it dry and chop it into small pieces. Prepare the vegetable stock with 600 ml hot water.
2. Sauté the onion and garlic in a pot with hot oil. Add the potato pieces and the carrot pieces. Fry briefly and add the vegetable stock. Season with salt, marjoram and pepper. Let the soup simmer for 25 minutes.
3. Puree the potato soup, season to taste and add seasoning if necessary. Heat the sausages in the soup and then serve the potato soup with two sausages each.

Turkey escalope with sage

Servings: 2

Level of difficulty: easy

Ingredients

- 2 turkey escalopes'
- 4 gr. sage leaves
- 2 slices Parma ham
- 1 paprika
- 2 carrots
- 300 g tomato pieces (tin)
- 2 tablespoons olive oil
- salt, pepper

Preparation

1. Rinse the meat and pat dry with kitchen towels. Beat the meat flat with a meat tenderizer.
2. Wash the peppers. Remove the stalk and core and then cut the peppers into strips. Peel the carrots and cut them into small rings. Wash the sage and shake dry.
3. Sprinkle the turkey escalope's with salt and pepper. Place 4 sage leaves and a slice of ham on each cutlet, roll up and fix with string.
4. Fry the turkey escalope's in a pan with hot oil. Then remove from the pan.
5. Add the vegetables to the pan and sauté. Season with salt and pepper. Add the chopped tomatoes and some water. Mix everything well. Put the meat back into the pan and cook for a quarter of an hour.
6. Serve the turkey escalopes with the vegetables. Serve with baguette.

Spaghetti Bolognese

Servings: 2

Level of difficulty: easy

Ingredients

- 250 g minced beef
- 140 g spaghetti
- ½ Onion
- 1 garlic clove
- 1 teaspoon tomato paste
- 300 g piece tomatoes (tin)
- salt, pepper

Preparation

1. Peel and chop the onion. Peel and chop the garlic.
2. Fry the onion and garlic in a pan with hot oil. Put the meat in the pan and fry it well. Season with salt and pepper.
3. Deglaze with 150 ml water after 5 minutes. Add the chunky tomatoes and the tomato paste and let everything simmer for about 20 minutes. Season to taste, adding salt and pepper if necessary.
4. Cook the pasta in salted water until al dente, drain and serve. Pour the Bolognese onto the pasta.

Optionally, you can also add half a chili pepper to the meat to give the dish a little spiciness.

Salmon with vegetables and rice

Servings: 2

Level of difficulty: easy

Ingredients

- 500 g saithe fillet (fresh or frozen)
- 250 Basmati wholemeal rice
- 1 each zucchini, paprika and eggplant
- 1 onion
- 1 garlic clove
- 2 tablespoons rapeseed oil
- 500 ml coconut milk
- salt, pepper

Preparation

1. Rinse the fish fillet, dab dry with kitchen paper and salt and pepper on both sides.
2. Peel and slice the zucchini. Wash the peppers. Remove the stalk and core and then cut the peppers into narrow strips. Wash the eggplant. Remove the stalk and then chop the eggplant. Peel and chop the onion. Peel and chop the garlic.
3. Cook the rice in salt water until al dente.
4. Sauté the onion and garlic in a pot with hot oil. Add the vegetables, season with salt and pepper and fry. Deglaze with the coconut milk.
5. Cut the fish into cubes and put them into the pot. Let everything cook for 5 minutes, season to taste and then serve.

Chicken Peanut Curry

Servings: 2

Level of difficulty: easy

Ingredients

- 200 g chicken breast
- 50 g peanuts
- 1 paprika
- ½ Chili
- 1 tablespoon fish sauce
- 200 ml coconut milk
- ½ tablespoons cane sugar
- 5 kefir leaves

Preparation

1. Wash the peppers. Remove the stalk and core and then cut the peppers into narrow strips.
2. Rinse the meat, dab dry with kitchen towel and cut into narrow strips.
3. Cut the chilies in half. Remove the seeds and the stalk.
4. Roast the peanuts in a pan without fat. Then remove and put aside.
5. Open the tin of coconut milk, take out the coconut oil and put it into the pan. Put the meat in the pan and fry for 3 minutes.
6. Add peanuts, peppers, chili and lime leaves to the pan. Mix everything well and simmer for 3 minutes. Then serve. Rice goes very well with this dish.

Zander with lenses

Servings: 2

Level of difficulty: easy

Ingredients

- 125 g belugal lentils
- 2 zander fillets (approx. 150 g each)
- 1 carrot
- 1 shallot
- 4 tablespoons olive oil
- Vegetable broth
- 2 stems of parsley
- salt, pepper

Preparation

1. Rinse the fish fillet, dab dry with kitchen paper and salt and pepper on both sides.
2. Peel the carrots and cut them into small slices. Wash the shallots. Remove the roots and cut the shallots into small rings. Prepare the vegetable stock with 300 ml hot water. Wash the parsley, shake it dry and chop it into small pieces. Mix the vegetable stock with 300 ml of hot water.
3. Sauté the shallots and carrot rings in a pan with hot oil. Add the lentils. Deglaze with the vegetable stock. Let everything simmer for a quarter of an hour.
4. In a pan with hot oil, fry the fish on both sides. Season with salt and pepper.
5. Serve the fish with the vegetables. Serve with rice.

Ribbon noodles with salmon and spinach

Servings: 2

Level of difficulty: easy

Ingredients

- 400 g wide ribbon noodles
- 2 salmon fillets (about 500 g)
- 500 g young spinach (Frozen)
- 250 g sour cream
- 2 tablespoons olive oil
- ½ Lemon
- salt, pepper

Preparation

1. Halve a lemon and squeeze one half. Collect the juice with a sieve in a cup. Rinse the fish fillet, dab dry with kitchen paper and salt and pepper on both sides. Defrost the spinach.
2. Sauté the spinach in a pan. Dice the fish and add to the spinach. Add the olive oil and sour cream, stir well and let everything simmer for 4 minutes. Season with salt, pepper and the lemon juice.
3. Cook the pasta in salted water until al dente, drain and serve. Serve the fish with the spinach.

Stuffed peppers

Servings: 2

Level of difficulty: easy

Ingredients

- 2 peppers
- 300 g minced meat
- 1 onion
- 1 garlic clove
- 1 tomato
- Vegetable broth
- one branch each of thyme and marjoram
- 1 tube of tomato paste
- 40 g breadcrumbs
- salt, pepper, olive oil, paprika powder (sweet)

Preparation

1. Wash the peppers. Cut off the lid of the peppers. Wash the tomato. Remove the stalk and then cut into small pieces.
2. Prepare the vegetable stock with 150 ml hot water.
3. Peel and chop the onion. Peel and chop the garlic.
4. Mix onion, garlic, breadcrumbs and meat. Pour the mixture into the peppers.
5. Fry the onion and garlic in a pan with hot oil.
6. Add the vegetable stock, the herbs, the diced tomatoes and some tomato paste to the pan. Stir well.
7. Add the peppers to the stock and simmer for three quarters of an hour. Then serve. Serve with rice or potatoes and some vegetables.

Saithe with fennel potatoes

Servings: 2

Level of difficulty: easy

Ingredients

- 2 pollack fillets (approx. 200 g each)
- 2 fennel tubers
- 250 g potatoes (floury cooking)
- 4 tablespoons of milk
- 50 g butter
- 1 lemon
- 1Tl fennel seed
- 1 sprig of thyme
- 4 tablespoons olive oil
- salt, pepper

Preparation

1. Peel potatoes, cut into small cubes and cook in salted water until al dente. Drain the water. Then press the potatoes through a potato press and mix them with the milk and butter.
2. Wash the thyme and shake dry.
3. Peel the fennel and chop into small pieces. Rinse the fish fillet, dab dry with kitchen paper and salt and pepper on both sides.
4. Put the fennel in an oven dish. Season with salt and pepper. Add thyme, fennel seeds and olive oil and cook the vegetables in the oven at 180 degrees for half an hour.
5. Sauté the fish in a pan with oil.
6. Place the fish fillets on plates, drizzle with lemon juice. Add the fennel and mashed potatoes.

Buddha Bowl

Servings: 2

Level of difficulty: easy

Ingredients

- 250 g chicken fillets
- 1 avocado
- 2 tablespoons peanuts
- 50 g baby spinach
- 2 limes
- 4 tablespoons olive oil
- salt, pepper

Preparation

1. Cut the avocado in half and use a spoon to lift the inside out of both halves and dice.
2. Roast the peanuts in a pan without fat.
3. Wash the chicken fillet, dab dry with kitchen paper, cut into wide strips and then fry vigorously on both sides in a pan with hot oil.
4. Cut the limes open. Squeeze the juice and collect it in a small bowl. Add 3 tablespoons of olive oil, salt and pepper.
5. Sauté the spinach, season and put it in two bowls. Add the meat, the avocado pieces and the roasted peanuts. Serve like this. Serve with the dressing.
6. If you like, you can also add quinoa and other vegetables.

Salmon easy and fast

Servings: 2

Level of difficulty: easy

Ingredients

- 2 salmon fillets (approx. 400 g)
- 1 tablespoon rapeseed oil
- 3 stems of parsley
- some lemon
- 1 baguette
- salt, pepper

Preparation

1. Rinse the fish fillet, dab dry with kitchen paper and salt and pepper on both sides. Wash the parsley, shake dry and chop finely.
2. Fry the salmon fillets in a pan with hot oil for 3 - 4 minutes. Turn the fish in half the time.
3. Bake a baguette in the oven.
4. Break the baguette in half and place one half on each plate. Add the fish, sprinkle with lemon and serve.
5. Serve with a fresh salad.

Linguine with mackerel

Servings: 2

Level of difficulty: easy

Ingredients

- 200 g linguine
- 2 mackerel fillets
- 1 shallot
- 1 stick of leek
- 100 ml cream
- Vegetable broth
- 1 tsp. mustard (hot)
- 2 stems dill

Preparation

1. Wash the dill, shake dry and chop finely. Wash the shallot and the leek. Remove the root base and cut both into small rings.
2. Put the shallots and the leeks into a coated pot. Place the fish on top of them.
3. Rinse the fish fillet, dab dry with kitchen paper, cut once lengthwise and once crosswise and place on the vegetables.
4. Prepare the vegetable stock with 50 ml of hot water, mix with mustard and cream and pour into the pot.
5. Put the lid on and cook the fish and vegetables for 5 minutes. Then take the fish out and keep it warm.
6. Cook the pasta in salted water until al dente and drain. Then fold into the vegetables. Simmer for a few minutes and serve with the fish.

Pork loin with spinach

Servings: 2

Level of difficulty: easy

Ingredients

- 2 slices pork loin
- 200 g young leaf spinach
- 100 g sheep's cheese
- 150 g potatoes (firm boiling)
- 1 onion
- 1 garlic clove
- salt, pepper

Preparation

1. Peel and chop the onion. Peel and chop the garlic.
2. Fry the onion and garlic in a pan with hot oil. Add the spinach and cook for 4 - 6 minutes. Season with salt and pepper.
3. Peel potatoes and cook them in salted water until al dente. Then drain the water and keep warm.
4. Sauté the meat in a pan with hot olive oil. Season with salt and pepper on both sides. Then continue to braise until it is done.
5. Serve the meat with the potatoes and spinach.

Sage Trout

Servings: 2

Level of difficulty: easy

Ingredients

- 2 trout (Frozen)
- 4 shallots
- 50 g clarified butter
- 250 ml apple juice
- 8 stems of sage
- 3 tablespoons flour
- salt, pepper

Preparation

1. Wash the shallots. Remove the root base and cut the shallots into small rings.
2. Rinse the fish fillets, dab dry with kitchen paper and salt and pepper them on both sides.
3. Melt the clarified butter in a pan. Add the trout and fry for 2 minutes on both sides. Then take the fillets out of the pan and keep them warm in the oven.
4. Add the shallots to the pan and sauté. After 5 minutes deglaze with the apple juice. Add the sage leaves and the flour. Mix everything well. Put the fish in the pan and cook with lid on for 12 minutes.
5. Serve the fish with the sauce and the shallots. Serve with rice or couscous.

Grilled salmon on cucumber salad

Servings: 2

Level of difficulty: easy

Ingredients

- 2 salmon fillets
- ½ Cucumber
- 1 spring onion
- 2 tablespoons olive oil
- 3 tsp soy sauce
- ½ tsp sesame oil
- mustard, pepper, salt, sugar

Preparation

1. Peel the cucumbers and cut into small rings. Put them into a bowl. Add soy sauce, sesame oil, salt, sugar, pepper and a little mustard. Mix everything well. Leave the salad to stand in the refrigerator for one hour.
2. Wash the spring onion. Remove the roots and cut the onion into small rings.
3. Rinse the fish filets, dab dry with kitchen paper and sprinkle salt and pepper on both sides.
4. Grill the salmon for 4 minutes on both sides, season with salt and pepper and place on a warm plate.
5. Put the cucumber salad on two plates and place the salmon on top. Serve like this.

Shrimps Asian

Servings: 2

Level of difficulty: easy

Ingredients

- 400 g prawns
- 125 g Basmati rice
- 1 avocado
- ½ Mango
- 2 tsp lemon juice
- ½ Chili
- 4 spring onions
- 3 tablespoons of oil
- ½ TL Curry
- salt, pepper

Preparation

1. Cut the avocado in half and use a spoon to lift the inside out of both halves. Sprinkle the pieces with lemon juice. Cut the mango in half. Remove the core and cut one half into small pieces. Put the other half in the refrigerator.
2. Wash the spring onions. Remove the roots and cut the onions into small rings. Rinse the prawns.
3. Cook the rice in salt water until al dente. Follow the packing instructions.
4. Sauté the prawns in hot oil. Season with salt and curry. Remove from the pan after 5 minutes.
5. Add the spring onions, rice and chilies to the pan. Fold in the mango and avocado. Steam for two minutes and then serve with the prawns.

Grilled trout

Servings: 2

Level of difficulty: easy

Ingredients

- 2 trouts
- 2 large potatoes (waxy)
- 500 g cream quark
- 2 lemons (organic)
- Garlic cloves
- ½ bunch of chives
- 4 sprigs thyme
- salt, pepper

Preparation

1. Wash the thyme and chives, shake dry and chop finely. Rinse the fish fillets and dab dry with kitchen paper. Then salt and pepper on both sides.
2. Peel potatoes, prick them with a fork and wrap them in aluminum foil. Then put them in the oven at 200 degrees for one hour.
3. Wash the lemon. Grate the peel and put it in a bowl. Add the quark. Season with salt and pepper. Mix everything well.
4. Fill the trout with the herbs, put them in a grill tongs and put them on the grill or oven for half an hour until the skin is crispy.
5. Take out the potatoes, cut them open and hollow them out with a spoon. Fill the quark into the opening and serve the potatoes this way. Add the fish.

Cod on ginger

Servings: 2

Level of difficulty: easy

Ingredients

- 2 cod fillets
- 250 g carrots
- 1 bunch of spring onions
- 1 red bell pepper
- ½ Lime
- 20 g ginger
- 3 tablespoons of oil
- Vegetable broth
- salt, pepper, some parsley

Preparation

1. Wash the spring onions. Remove the roots and cut the onions into small rings. Peel the carrots and cut them into small slices. Wash the peppers. Remove the stalk and core and then cut the peppers into small strips. Prepare the vegetable stock with 100 ml of hot water. Peel and grate the ginger.
2. Rinse the fish fillets and pat dry with kitchen paper. Then salt and pepper on both sides and fry them in a pan with hot oil for 10 minutes. Turn the fillets over in half the time. Remove the fish from the pan and keep it warm in the oven.
3. Sauté the ginger with the carrots and peppers in a pan with hot oil. Season with salt and pepper and serve with the fish.

Cod on pumpkin

Servings: 2

Level of difficulty: easy

Ingredients

- 2 cod fillets
- 600 g pumpkin
- 250 g leek
- 1 chili
- 20 g ginger
- 1 lime
- 200 ml coconut milk
- 100 ml vegetable broth
- salt, oil

Preparation

1. Cook the pumpkin for 3 minutes in the microwave on 600 watts, open, take out the flesh and cut into large pieces. Peel and grate the ginger. Wash the leeks, remove the roots and remove the outer leaf, then cut into small rings.
2. Wash the lime with hot water. Grate the peel. Divide the lime and squeeze out the juice and catch it.
3. Sauté the pumpkin. Add the leek and half of the ginger and half of the chili. Stir well. Deglaze with the lime juice, coconut milk and vegetable stock and simmer for 6 minutes.
4. Chop the chilies into small pieces and crush them in a mortar with the lime zest and ginger. Rub the resulting paste into the fish fillets.
5. Fry the fish in hot oil for 3 minutes on both sides and serve. Add the vegetables.

Golden trout with salad

Servings: 2

Level of difficulty: easy

Ingredients

- 2 gold trout (220 g each)
- 500 g potatoes
- ½ Lemon
- 150 g lamb's lettuce
- 1 tablespoon of clarified butter
- 1 tablespoon safflower oil
- 2 tablespoons butter
- salt, pepper

Preparation

1. Peel potatoes and cook them in salted water until al dente. Drain the water afterwards.
2. Sort the lamb's lettuce, wash and shake dry. (Watch out for stones!)
3. Rinse the fish fillets and pat dry with kitchen paper. Then salt and pepper on both sides and fry them in a pan with hot clarified butter for 14 minutes. Turn the fillets over in half the time. Remove the fish from the pan and keep it warm in the oven.
4. Cut the lemon in half. Put one half aside and squeeze the other. In a small bowl mix lemon juice with safflower oil, salt and pepper to a dressing.
5. Serve the fish. Add the salad and keep the dressing handy.

Ham noodles

Servings: 2

Level of difficulty: easy

Ingredients

- 200 g ham (cooked)
- Vegetable broth
- 1 pack of processed cheese
- Spice mixture
- 300 g wholemeal noodles

Preparation

1. Prepare the vegetable stock with 250 ml hot water. Put it into a pot, heat it up and dissolve the processed cheese in it.
2. Dice the ham and put it in the pot
3. Cook the pasta in salted water until al dente, drain and serve. Pour the ham and cheese sauce over it.

Hearty omelet

Servings: 2

Level of difficulty: easy

Ingredients

- 4 eggs
- 50 ml milk
- ½ Onion
- 4 slices of salami
- 2 tablespoons hard cheese
- Oil

Preparation

1. Peel and chop the onion. Grate the hard cheese.
2. Beat the eggs and put them into a bowl. Add the milk. Chop the salami and add it to the egg milk. Mix everything well.
3. Heat the oil in a frying pan and fry the omelets.
4. Serve the omelet with a fresh salad and a baguette.

Vegan kitchen

Green beans with mushrooms

Servings: 2

Level of difficulty: easy

Ingredients

- 125 g chanterelles (alternatively mushrooms)
- 500 g green beans
- 3 sprigs savory
- 1 onion
- 2 garlic cloves
- 1 tablespoon butter
- salt, pepper, sugar

Preparation

1. Peel and chop the onion. Peel and chop the garlic.
2. Wash the savory and shake dry.
3. Sort the mushrooms, clean and chop them. Rinse the mushrooms from the glass and cut them into small pieces.
4. Cut off the ends of the beans, wash the beans and cut them into pieces about 2 cm long. Boil them in a pot with salted water and the savory. After 10 minutes remove from the heat and drain.
5. Fry the onion in a pan with hot butter until golden brown. Add the garlic and the mushrooms. Season with salt, a pinch of sugar and pepper.
6. Add the beans to the pan and fry for a few minutes. Season to taste and if necessary, add salt and pepper.
7. Place on two plates, garnish with fresh herbs and serve.

Broccoli with nuts

Servings: 2

Level of difficulty: easy

Ingredients

- 400 g broccoli
- 2 tablespoons walnut kernels
- Vegetable broth
- 1 onion
- 1 tablespoon lemon juice
- ½ tablespoons of nut oil (or olive oil)
- salt, pepper

Preparation

1. Chop the walnut kernels into small pieces. Prepare the vegetable stock with 150 ml hot water. Peel and chop the onion. Wash the broccoli and divide into small florets. Cut off the stems.
2. Roast the nuts in a coated pan without fat.
3. Put the vegetable broth in a pan, heat it up and when it boils, add the broccoli. Let it simmer for about 4 - 6 minutes and then drain. Collect the broccoli stock.
4. Mix lemon juice, oil, onion and broccoli stock. Season with salt and pepper.
5. Arrange the broccoli on flat plates. Pour the broccoli stock over it and sprinkle the nuts on top.

Chinese cabbage rolls

Servings: 2

Level of difficulty: easy

Ingredients

- 1 Chinese cabbage (approx. 200 g)
- 4 dried apricots
- 100 g natural rice
- 1 tsp curry powder
- Butter
- 5 g egg substitute (Bio vegan egg substitute vegetable)
- Vegetable broth
- Salt

Preparation

1. Prepare the vegetable stock with 75 ml hot water. Chop the apricots finely. Clean the Chinese cabbage.
2. Preheat the oven to 200 degrees (circulating air).
3. Cook the rice in salt water. Add the apricots and curry to the rice. Reduce heat, put lid on and simmer the apricot rice for three quarters of an hour.
4. Grease a casserole dish. Blanch 8 leaves of Chinese cabbage and then lay them out on a work board.
5. Cut the remaining cabbage into small pieces and add to the rice. Mix the egg replacer with 50 ml water and add it. Mix everything well and pile up on the cabbage leaves.
6. Roll up the leaves. Fix them with white string or roulade needles and then put them into the baking tin. Put them in the oven for half an hour and serve. Serve with a fresh salad,

Endive mashed potatoes

Servings: 2

Level of difficulty: easy

Ingredients

- 800 g potatoes (floury cooking)
- 350 g endive salad
- 2 tablespoons of oil
- 200 ml soy milk
- 1 onion
- Nutmeg
- salt, pepper

Preparation

1. Peel potatoes, cut into small cubes and cook in salted water until al dente. Then drain the water and put the potatoes in a large bowl.
2. Sort the endive salad, wash and shake dry.
3. Peel and chop the onion. Sauté the onion in a pan with hot oil. Add the salad to the pan.
4. Mash the potatoes. Bring the soy milk to the boil and add it to the mashed potatoes. Add the endive mixture. Season with salt and pepper. Season to taste, add salt and pepper if necessary and serve.

Risotto with radicchio

Servings: 2

Level of difficulty: easy

Ingredients

- 100 g risotto rice
- Vegetable broth
- 1 head radicchio
- 1 apple
- 4 tablespoons vegan parmesan (grated)
- salt, pepper

Preparation

1. Prepare the vegetable stock with 500 ml hot water.
2. Clean the radicchio. Wash the leaves. Remove the stalk.
3. Peel the apple. Remove the core and the stem base and then cut the apple into narrow slices.
4. Sauté the rice in a pot with hot rape seed oil. Deglaze with the vegetable stock, cover and simmer for 25 minutes.
5. Add the apple pieces, the radicchio and the parmesan to the rice.
6. Season with salt and pepper.
7. Season to taste, if necessary, season with salt and pepper and serve.

Beet with walnut

Servings: 2

Level of difficulty: easy

Ingredients

- 600 g beet
- 40 g walnut kernels
- 150 g vegan low-fat curd cheese
- 7 tablespoons orange juice
- 1 tablespoon of mustard
- 2 tablespoons olive oil
- salt, pepper

Preparation

1. Preheat the oven to 200 degrees (circulating air).
1. Chop the walnut kernels into small pieces. Cover a baking tray with baking paper.
2. Peel the beetroot, cut it into small cubes and put it on the baking tray. Sprinkle salt and pepper over it. Put the beetroot in the oven for three quarters of an hour.
3. Roast the nuts in a coated pan without fat.
4. Mix in the quark. Mix in the nuts. Season to taste and add salt and pepper if necessary.
5. Mix the orange juice in a small bowl with the mustard, salt and pepper to a dressing.
6. Place the beetroot on a plate. Layer the curd mixture on top and pour the dressing over it.

Red cabbage with pear

Servings: 2

Level of difficulty: easy

Ingredients

- 600 g red cabbage
- 1 onion
- ½ tablespoons rapeseed oil
- 2 tablespoons wild berries (glass)
- 1 bay leaf
- 1 clove
- Vegetable broth
- 1 bulb
- 1 tablespoon red wine vinegar
- salt, pepper

Preparation

1. Peel and chop the onion. Mix the vegetable stock with 200 ml hot water. Remove the outer leaves from the red cabbage. Cut the cabbage open. Cut out the stalk. Chop the cabbage and wash it.
2. Sauté the onion in a pan with hot oil. Add the cabbage. After 6 minutes add the wild berries, the bay leaf, the cloves and the vegetable broth. Cover and simmer for 20 min.
3. Peel the pear. Remove the core and the stem base and then cut the pear into small pieces. Add these to the cabbage and steam for 10 minutes. Season to taste and serve the dish.

Asparagus packages

Servings: 2

Level of difficulty: easy

Ingredients

- 1 kg asparagus
- 4 tablespoons Rama (or Alsan organic)
- salt, pepper

Preparation

1. Preheat the oven to 200 degrees (circulating air).
2. Peel the asparagus, cut off the ends and then cut the asparagus into small pieces about 1 - 2 cm long.
3. Lay out 4 large pieces of aluminum foil and spread the asparagus on top.
4. Season the asparagus with salt and pepper. Divide the rama into four roughly equal parts and place them on the asparagus packets. Fold the aluminum foil into packages and place them on a baking tray.
5. Bake the asparagus parcels for 50 minutes and serve immediately. Serve with parsley potatoes.

Turnip ramming

Servings: 2

Level of difficulty: easy

Ingredients

- 400 g rutabaga (approx. ½ turnip)
- 2 garlic cloves
- 1 lemon
- 2 tablespoons rapeseed oil
- 1 tablespoon of sugar
- 100 ml soy cooking cream
- salt, pepper

Preparation

1. Preheat the oven to 200 degrees (circulating air).
2. Squeeze the lemon. Collect the juice with a sieve in a cup. Peel and chop the garlic. Peel the turnip, cut it into small cubes and put it in a bowl.
3. Add the garlic, rapeseed oil, lemon juice and sugar to the beet. Mix everything well.
4. Cover a baking tray with aluminum foil and apply the mixture. Cook these 50 min in the oven.
5. Let the mixture cool down a bit, put it into a pot, add the cooking cream, salt and pepper and puree everything finely. Then warm it up again and serve.
6. Add mashed potatoes, a light chasseur sauce and a fresh salad.

Tomato rice

Servings: 2

Level of difficulty: easy

Ingredients

- 400 g tomatoes
- 1 stick of leek
- 2 garlic cloves
- 300 g long grain rice
- 1 tablespoon of oil
- Vegetable broth
- salt, pepper
- 50 g vegan cheese spread

Preparation

1. Prepare the vegetable stock with 400 ml hot water.
2. Wash the leeks. Remove the roots and cut the onions into small rings.
3. Peel and chop the garlic.
4. Wash the tomatoes. Remove the stalk and then cut the tomatoes into small pieces.
5. Sauté the leek and garlic in a pan with hot oil.
6. Add the rice, steam for a few minutes and then deglaze with the vegetable broth.
7. Add the tomato pieces. Season with salt and pepper. Mix everything well and let simmer covered for 20 minutes.
8. Grate the hard cheese and add it to the tomato rice. Season to taste, adding salt and pepper if necessary and then serve. Serve with a fresh salad.

Fennel, braised

Servings: 2

Level of difficulty: easy

Ingredients

- 2 fennel tubers (approx. 500 g)
- 2 tomatoes
- 2 shallots
- 2 garlic cloves
- 2 sprigs thyme
- 2 tablespoons olive oil
- salt, pepper, sugar

Preparation

1. Wash the tomatoes. Remove the stalk and cut the tomatoes into small pieces.
2. Wash the shallots. Remove the roots and cut the onions into small rings.
3. Peel and chop the garlic.
4. Peel the fennel and chop into small pieces.
5. Wash the thyme, shake dry and chop finely.
6. Sauté the shallots, garlic and thyme in a pan with hot oil.
7. Add tomatoes and fennel. Season with salt, some sugar and pepper.
8. Put the lid on and let everything simmer for 20 minutes.
9. Season to taste, if necessary, season with salt and pepper and serve.

Leek with marinade

Servings: 2

Level of difficulty: easy

Ingredients

- 500 g leek
- Vegetable broth
- ¼ TL coriander seeds
- 3 allspice grains
- 1 bay leaf
- 3 sprigs thyme
- 1 tablespoon lemon juice
- 2 tablespoons olive oil

Preparation

1. Prepare the vegetable stock with 500 ml hot water. Wash the thyme, shake dry and chop finely.
2. Clean and wash the leeks, remove the stalk and then cut them into rings.
3. Put the vegetable stock in a pot and heat it up. When it boils, add coriander, allspice, bay leaf and thyme. Add the leek pieces to the mixture and let it simmer for 6 - 8 minutes.
4. Lift out the leek. Mix vinegar, lemon juice and olive oil in a bowl. Add some 250 ml of the vegetable stock.
5. Pour the sauce over the leek and leave it in the refrigerator for 2 hours. Then warm it up in the oven and serve.
6. Rice or couscous, a fresh paprika salad and a few vegetable meatballs go well with it.

Brussels sprout gratin

Servings: 2

Level of difficulty: easy

Ingredients

- 600 g Brussels sprouts
- 1 onion
- 100 g Gouda (air-dried vegan Gouda, or bedda Block classic)
- 1 sprig of thyme
- 400 ml milk
- 20 g egg substitute (Bio vegan egg substitute vegetable)
- Spaetzle

Preparation

1. Wash the thyme, shake dry and chop finely.
2. Peel and chop the onion.
3. Grate the Gouda finely.
4. Sort the sprouts, remove the outer leaves that are no longer good. Wash the sprouts and then cut the florets in half.
5. Preheat the oven to 200 degrees (circulating air).
6. Cook the brussels sprouts in a pot with salted water until al dente. Pour off the water with a sieve, mix with onion and spaetzle and put into an oven dish.
7. Mix the milk, egg substitute, thyme, salt and pepper and place on the Brussels sprouts. Sprinkle the cheese on top.
8. Bake the Brussels sprouts for three quarters of an hour and serve immediately.
9. If you like, you can also add some ham to the mixture.

Wraps with rocket and carrot

Servings: 2

Level of difficulty: easy

Ingredients

- Organic coconut wraps
- 1 handful of rocket
- 6 tablespoons ricotta
- 1 carrot
- salt, pepper

Preparation

1. Sort the rocket, wash and shake dry.
2. Peel the carrot and cut into small rings.
3. Lay out release paper. Place the wraps on top.
4. Put the rocket on the wraps and the carrot pieces on top.
5. Put the ricotta on top.
6. Sprinkle some salt and pepper on the tortillas and roll them up.

Baked potatoes

Servings: 2

Level of difficulty: easy

Ingredients

- 2 potatoes (large, firm boiling)
- fresh herbs (mixture or fresh different, depending on taste)
- Olive oil
- Salt
- Vegan quark (made from soybeans, almonds or cashew nuts)

Preparation

1. Preheat the oven to 200 degrees (circulating air).
2. Cover a baking tray with baking paper.
3. Peel the potatoes, cut them in half and put them on the baking paper. The cut open flat side should face upwards.
4. Brush the potatoes with oil. Sprinkle the salt and the herbs. Then bake the potatoes for three quarters of an hour.
5. Very well fits coarse sea salt and rosemary that you sprinkle on the potatoes. Serve the baked potatoes with a fresh salad and homemade herb quark.

Potato and carrot vegetables

Servings: 2

Level of difficulty: easy

Ingredients

- 250 g potatoes (mainly waxy)
- 500 g carrots
- ½ Vegetable onion
- 1 ½ Garlic cloves
- Vegetable broth
- 1 oil
- ½ tablespoons of flour
- salt, pepper

Preparation

1. Prepare the vegetable stock with 500 ml hot water. Peel potatoes, cut into small cubes and cook in salted water until firm to the bite. Drain the water and put the potatoes in a large bowl. Peel the carrots and cut them into small slices. Peel and chop the onion.
2. Pour the vegetable stock into a pot. Add the carrots and garlic, bring to the boil and simmer for a quarter of an hour at reduced heat.
3. Add the potatoes and simmer until they are done. Drain the broth and take the pot off the heat.
4. Mix oil and flour in a frying pan to make a roux. Add the vegetables. Season with salt and pepper. And let it simmer for a few minutes.
5. Season to taste, if necessary, season with salt and pepper and serve. Serve with a fresh salad.

Zucchini ribbon noodles

Servings: 2

Level of difficulty: easy

Ingredients

- 250 g ribbon noodles
- 350 g zucchini
- 1 onion
- 108 g (Bio vegan whipping cream)
- 3 saffron threads
- 30 g Rama
- 3 tablespoons vegan Parmesan (freshly grated, e.g. Jeezano block hard melt, Violife Prosociano corner)
- salt, pepper

Preparation

1. Peel and chop the onion. Peel and slice the zucchini. Cook the noodles in salted water until they are firm to the bite. Then drain the water.
2. Sauté the onion in a pan with hot oil. Add the zucchini to the pan. Season with salt and pepper. Add cream and saffron. Mix well and simmer for a few minutes.
3. Serve the zucchini vegetables with the noodles. Sprinkle the Parmesan cheese over it.

Brussels sprouts classic

Servings: 2
Level of difficulty: easy

Ingredients

- 500 g Brussels sprouts
- 1 onion (small)
- Oil
- ¼ tsp sugar
- Nutmeg
- Vegetable broth
- 3 stems of parsley
- salt, pepper

Preparation

1. Peel and chop the onion. Sort the brussels sprouts, remove the outer leaves that are no longer good.
2. Wash the parsley, shake dry and chop finely.
3. Wash the sprouts and then cut the florets in half. Cook the sprouts in a pot with salted water until al dente. Drain the water with a sieve.
4. Prepare the vegetable stock with 30 ml hot water.
5. Sauté the onion in a pot with hot oil. Add sugar.
6. Add the Brussels sprouts to the pan. Season with salt, nutmeg and pepper. Mix everything well and simmer for 8 minutes.
7. Add the vegetable stock and simmer everything for another 10 minutes. Serve Ann. Sprinkle the parsley over the Brussels sprouts.

Potato Snow

Servings: 2

Level of difficulty: easy

Ingredients

- 450 g potatoes
- 5 stems dill
- Olive Oil
- Salt

Preparation

1. Wash the dill, shake dry and chop finely.
2. Peel potatoes and cook them in salted water until al dente. Then drain the water and put the potatoes in a large bowl.
3. Press the potatoes through a potato press.
4. Add olive oil to the potatoes. Sprinkle on the dill. Serve the potatoes.
5. Serve with fried vegetables and a fresh salad.

Spinach Sicilian style

Servings: 2

Level of difficulty: easy

Ingredients

- 400 g leaf spinach
- 30 g raisins
- 3 garlic cloves
- 30 g pine nuts
- 1 lemon
- salt, pepper, nutmeg

Preparation

1. Wash, sort and chop the spinach. Peel and chop the garlic.
2. Fry the pine nuts in a pan with hot oil. Add the garlic.
3. Add the spinach to the pan and fry for 5 minutes.
4. Add raisins, salt, pepper and nutmeg. Mix well, season to taste and serve.
5. The potato snow goes very well with it.

Mushrooms in Balsamic

Servings: 2

Level of difficulty: easy

Ingredients

- 425 g mushrooms mixed
- 2 stems of parsley
- 2 garlic cloves
- Vegetable broth
- 3 tablespoons balsamic vinegar
- 2 tablespoons olive oil
- salt, pepper

Preparation

1. Sort the mushrooms, clean and chop them. Rinse the mushrooms from the glass and cut them into small pieces.
2. Wash the parsley, shake dry and chop finely. Peel and chop the garlic. Prepare the vegetable stock with 251750 ml hot water.
3. Sauté the garlic in a pan with hot oil. Add the mushrooms to the pan. Season with salt and pepper. Fry the mushrooms for 5 minutes.
4. Deglaze with the vegetable stock. Add parsley and balsamic vinegar. Stir well and let everything simmer for 4 minutes. Season to taste, add salt and pepper if necessary and serve. Serve with a fresh salad.

Marinated zucchinis

Servings: 2

Level of difficulty: easy

Ingredients

- 3 zucchinis (about 750 g)
- 3 stems of mint
- 2 tablespoons honey
- 2 tablespoons olive oil
- salt, pepper

Preparation

1. Wash the mint, shake dry and chop finely.
2. Peel and slice the zucchini.
3. Put the mint in a small bowl. Add oil, honey and lemon juice. Mix everything well.
4. Spread the zucchini slices with the oil mixture (or put them briefly in it) and then put the slices on the grill. Grill the slices for 3 minutes on each side and then serve.
5. Other grilled foods such as corn on the cob or vegetable skewers and a fresh salad are sufficient.

Italian style oven vegetables

Servings: 2

Level of difficulty: easy

Ingredients

- 2 peppers (red and yellow)
- 1 fennel bulb
- 2 carrots
- 2 onions
- 3 tablespoons olive oil
- 2 stems each of basil and oregano
- Balsamic vinegar
- salt, pepper

Preparation

1. Preheat the oven to 200 degrees (circulating air).
2. Wash the peppers. Remove the stalk and core and then cut the peppers into narrow strips. Peel the carrots and cut them into small slices. Peel and chop the onion. Wash the herbs, shake dry and chop finely. Peel the fennel and cut into small cubes.
3. Put the vegetables in a bowl. Add the olive oil, salt and pepper.
4. Cover a baking tray with baking paper. Layer the vegetables on top. Put them in the oven for half an hour.
5. Sprinkle the oven vegetables with herbs when serving. Baked potatoes, potato snow, fried potatoes, rosemary potatoes or similar go well with it. Refine with balsamic vinegar as required.

Pumpkin fryers

Servings: 2

Level of difficulty: easy

Ingredients

- 100 g pumpkin
- 200 g chick peas (tinned, frozen or fresh)
- 1 onion
- ½ garlic clove
- 3 tablespoons chickpea flour
- 1 tablespoon breadcrumbs
- salt, pepper

Preparation

1. Rinse the chickpeas and cook them in a pot of salted water until al dente. Then drain the water and put the chickpeas aside.
2. Peel the pumpkin. Remove the core. Cut the flesh into small pieces. We only need 100 g. Put the remaining pumpkin aside.
3. Peel and chop the onion. Peel and chop the garlic.
4. Put the pumpkin, chickpeas, onions and garlic in a large mixing bowl and puree. Put the mixture into a bowl. Season with salt and pepper. Add breadcrumbs and chickpea flour.
5. Shape the dough into small flat roasts and fry them vigorously on both sides in a pan with hot oil. Serve the still warm roastings. Serve with mashed potatoes, fried vegetables and a fresh salad.

Caprese with beans

Servings: 2

Level of difficulty: easy

Ingredients

- 2 tomatoes
- 1 Mozzarella (Mozzarisella von Frescolat)
- 150 g green beans
- 3 tablespoons olive oil
- 3 tablespoons balsamic vinegar
- 1 teaspoon rice syrup
- 1 sprig of thyme
- 1 teaspoon mustard

Preparation

1. Wash the tomatoes. Remove the stalk and then cut the tomatoes into small slices. Cut the mozzarella into slices as well. Wash the thyme, shake dry and chop finely. Cut off the ends of the beans, wash the beans and cut them into pieces about 2 cm long.
2. Cook the beans in a pan with hot oil for 10 minutes. Season with salt, thyme and pepper.
3. Layer tomato slices and mozzarella on two plates. Alternate slices of tomato and cheese. Leave the center free.
4. Put olive oil in a bowl. Add balsamic vinegar, rice syrup, mustard, salt and pepper. Mix everything thoroughly and put it on the cheese and tomato slices.
5. Place the beans in the middle of the plates and serve.

Tofu vegetables

Servings: 2

Level of difficulty: easy

Ingredients

- 100 g tofu
- 1 onion
- 1 zucchini
- 2 eggplants
- 1 carrot
- 2 tablespoons olive oil
- 3 stems thyme
- salt, pepper

Preparation

1. Preheat the oven to 200 degrees (circulating air).
2. Cover a baking tray with baking paper.
3. Cut the tofu into cubes. Peel and chop the onion. Peel and slice the zucchini. Peel the carrot and cut into small rings. Wash the eggplant. Remove the steep part and then dice the eggplant. Wash the thyme, shake dry and chop finely.
4. Put the vegetables on the baking tray. Drizzle the olive oil. Sprinkle with salt, pepper and the thyme and then bake the vegetables for three quarters of an hour.
5. Serve the vegetables with the tofu fresh from the oven. Serve with couscous, rice, noodles or rosemary potatoes.

Paprika Pasta

Servings: 2

Level of difficulty: easy

Ingredients

- 3 Peppers (colored)
- ½ Onion
- 1 garlic clove
- 5 basil leaves
- 100 g Mascarpone (Crème)
- 2 tsp lemon juice
- salt, pepper
- 300 g pasta

Preparation

1. Preheat the oven to 200 degrees (circulating air).
2. Wash the peppers. Peel the onion. Peel and chop the garlic. Pluck the basil leaves, wash and dry them with kitchen paper.
3. Brush the bell pepper and onion with oil and roast in the oven for half an hour.
4. Let the paprika and onion cool down a little, then cut them into small pieces and mix them with the basil leaves in a mixing bowl.
5. Add garlic, mascarpone and lemon juice to the blender jug and puree. Pour the finished paste into a bowl and season with salt and pepper.
6. Cook the pasta in salted water until al dente, drain and serve. Serve with the pasta.

Chili Tomato Ribbon Noodles

Servings: 2

Level of difficulty: easy

Ingredients

- 200 g cocktail tomatoes
- 10 g coriander (fresh)
- 1 spring onion
- 1 chili
- 2 tablespoons tomato paste
- 1 teaspoon olive oil (or butter)
- 300 g ribbon noodles
- Pepper

Preparation

1. Wash and quarter the cocktail tomatoes. Wash the coriander, shake dry and chop into small pieces. Chop the chilies. Remove the stalk and the seeds.
2. Cook the pasta in salted water until al dente and drain. Stir some olive oil into the noodles (or butter).
3. Pour the cocktail tomatoes into a mixer. Add coriander, spring onions and chili. Puree everything well and fill into a bowl. Add the tomato paste. Season the salsa with pepper and season to taste.
4. Serve the pasta with the salsa.

Swiss chard curry

Servings: 2

Level of difficulty: easy

Ingredients

- 300 g chard
- ½ Onion
- 1 garlic clove
- 1 sweet potato (approx. 200 g)
- 125 g wild rice
- 75 g mountain lentils
- 2 tablespoons rapeseed oil
- 200 ml coconut milk
- some curry
- salt, pepper

Preparation

1. Wash, clean and chop the chard.
2. Peel and chop the onion. Peel and chop the garlic. Peel the potato and cut it into small cubes. Rinse the lentils and prepare them according to the package label. Cook the rice in salt water until al dente.
3. Fry the onion and garlic in a pan with hot oil.
4. Add the potato to the pan and fry for 5 minutes. Season with salt and pepper. Add the chard and fry everything for another 5 minutes.
5. Add the curry and the coconut milk to the pan. Mix everything well and simmer for 5 minutes. Add the lentils to the mixture. Season to taste and then serve with the rice.

Rocket-lemon pesto with noodles

Servings: 2

Level of difficulty: easy

Ingredients

- 110 g rocket salad
- 1 garlic clove
- 150 g cocktail tomatoes
- 50 pine nuts
- 50 ml olive oil
- ½ Organic lemon
- salt, pepper
- 300 g pasta

Preparation

1. Wash and quarter the cocktail tomatoes. Sort the rocket, wash and shake dry. Peel and chop the garlic.
2. Roast the pine nuts in a pan without fat.
3. Wash the lemon, halve it and squeeze one half. Then grate the peel.
4. Place the cocktail tomatoes in a mixing bowl. Add the garlic pieces, the pine nuts, the grated lemon, the lemon juice and the olive oil. Mix everything well and place in a bowl. Season with salt and pepper.
5. Cook the pasta in salted water until al dente, drain and serve. Serve with the pesto.

Sweets &

Desserts

Tofu Chocolate Mouse

Servings: 2

Level of difficulty: easy

Ingredients

- 100 g dark chocolate (cocoa content 70%)
- 1 organic orange
- 1 vanilla pod
- 80 g coconut blossom sugar
- 700 g silk tofu
- 40 g cocoa
- 3 tablespoons of espresso (cooled down)
- 20 g chickpea flour
- 100 ml soy milk
- Salt

Preparation

1. Mix the egg replacer with 100 ml water.
2. Wash the orange with hot water. Rub off the peel.
3. Scrape out the vanilla pod. Mix the pulp with the coconut blossom sugar.
4. Place the tofu in a bowl and mix with the cocoa, orange zest, vanilla coconut blossom sugar and espresso.
5. Melt the chocolate in a water bath and then add it to the tofu. Mix everything well.
6. Mix the chickpea flour with 100 ml soy milk, add a pinch of salt and fold into the tofu. Pour the finished mouse into two glasses and serve.

Berry Biscuit Trifle

Servings: 2

Level of difficulty: easy

Ingredients

- 150 g quark (fat content: 20%)
- 150 g yoghurt
- 300 g berry mixture (raspberries, blueberries, strawberries, depending on the offer and season, fresh or frozen)
- 1 tablespoon honey
- 1 pinch of cinnamon
- 6 wholemeal oat cookies

Preparation

1. Place the curd in a bowl. Add the yoghurt and honey and a little cinnamon. Mix everything together well.
2. Select and wash the berries. Remove small remaining stalks. Defrost the frozen goods.
3. Place the cookies on a plate and crush them.
4. Fill in two glasses layer by layer and alternately the quark yoghurt mixture, the crushed cookies and the berries. Serve the mixture in this way.

Apricot Mouse

Servings: 2

Level of difficulty: easy

Ingredients

- 200 g apricots
- 50 ml apple juice
- 1 package of vanilla sugar
- 200 g quark (fat content: 20%)
- 150 g yoghurt (fat content: 1.5%)
- 1 tablespoon honey
- 1 tablespoon of poppy seeds (who likes can also use sesame seeds)

Preparation

1. Wash the apricots, cut them in half and remove the stone.
2. Put an apricot aside. Chop the others and put them in a blender. Add the apple juice and puree everything well. Mix the vanilla sugar into the puree.
3. Put the quark in a bowl and mix with the yogurt, honey and poppy seeds.
4. Fill in two glasses layer by layer and alternately the quark yoghurt mixture and the apricot puree. Serve the mixture in this way.
5. Place half an apricot on top of each jar.

Plum with cinnamon cream

Servings: 2

Level of difficulty: easy

Ingredients

- 300 g plums
- 1 tsp butter
- 2 tablespoons cane sugar
- 50 ml apple juice
- 1 capsule cardamom
- 1 anisotropic star
- 50 ml cream

Preparation

1. Wash the plums, cut them in half and remove the stone.
2. Melt the butter in a pan. Add the plums and sauté a little. Add 1 tablespoon cane sugar and let it caramelize.
3. Use the apple juice to deglaze. Add the cardamom and the aniseed star and let the mixture simmer for 10 minutes.
4. Fish the spices from the pan. Remove the plums from the heat and let them cool down.
5. Pour the plums into jars or compote bowls.
6. Mix the cream with 1 tablespoon cane sugar, whip until stiff and then place on top of the plums.
7. **To be observed**: Season dishes only with little or no cinnamon. The consumption of too much cinnamon can possibly trigger contractions. Therefore, you should only season dishes during pregnancy with a pinch of cinnamon or avoid cinnamon altogether.

Fruit salad with sea buckthorn

Servings: 2

Level of difficulty: easy

Ingredients

- 100 g pineapple (tin)
- 100 g mango
- 100 g papaya
- 1 banana
- 1 tablespoon hazelnuts
- 1 tablespoon coconut flakes
- 2 tablespoons orange juice
- 1 tablespoon sea buckthorn concentrate (from the health food store)

Preparation

1. Peel the mango and papaya and cut 100 g of the fruit into small pieces.
2. Peel and slice the banana.
3. Put the fruits in a large bowl.
4. Add the hazelnuts, coconut flakes, orange juice and sea buckthorn concentrate.
5. Mix everything well, pour into two bowls and serve.

Berry-Almond Crumble

Servings: 2

Level of difficulty: easy

Ingredients

- 300 g berry mixture (raspberries, blueberries, strawberries, depending on the offer and season, fresh or frozen)
- 70 g wholemeal flour
- 150 g yoghurt
- 20 g almonds
- 40 g cane sugar
- 40 g butter
- 1 pinch of salt
- 1 package vanilla sugar

Preparation

1. Preheat the oven to 200 degrees (circulating air).
2. Select and wash the berries. Use frozen food, defrost them.
3. Put the berries in an oven dish.
4. Put the flour in a bowl. Add almonds, sugar, butter and salt and mix well. Pour the resulting crumbled dough on the berries.
5. Bake the crumble in the oven for half an hour.
6. Cut the crumble while still warm and put it on plates.
7. Mix the yoghurt with the vanilla sugar and pour it onto the crumble. Serve like this.

Vanilla ice cream homemade

Servings: 2

Level of difficulty: easy

Ingredients

- 50 g cashew nuts
- 6 dates (dried, without stone)
- ½ TL Vanilla
- 1 pinch of salt
- 200 ml milk

Preparation

1. Cut the dates into small pieces.
2. Chop the cashew nuts into small pieces.
3. Put both in a blender with the vanilla and salt.
4. Add 200 ml milk.
5. Mix the mixture, fill it into ice molds and put it in the freezer.

Buckwheat pancakes

Servings: 2

Level of difficulty: easy

Ingredients

- 140 g buckwheat flour
- 125 g raspberries (fresh or frozen)
- 1 tablespoon rice syrup
- 1 egg
- 100 ml milk
- 100 ml mineral water
- 1 teaspoon baking powder
- 1 pinch of salt
- Oil

Preparation

1. Mix the flour with the baking powder and an egg. Add the rice syrup, milk and water.
2. Mix everything together well. Let the dough rest for ten minutes.
3. Take the dough out of the bowl with a small ladle and bake it in a pan with hot oil. Use a spatula to turn the pancakes.
4. Select and wash the raspberries. Remove small remaining stems. Mix the berries to a puree and apply it to the pancakes. Serve them like this.

Puffed rice with chocolate

Servings: 2

Level of difficulty: easy

Ingredients

- 100 g dark chocolate (cocoa content: 70%)
- 30 g quinoa (puffed)
- 2 tablespoons peanut puree / peanut butter (or add a few finely chopped nuts)
- 2 tablespoons peanuts

Preparation

1. Chop the peanuts finely.
2. Melt the chocolate in a water bath.
3. Stir the peanut purée into the chocolate. Mix the two together well.
4. Fold the puffed quinoa and peanuts into the chocolate.
5. Spread out a piece of baking paper and pour on the chocolate mixture. Put it in the refrigerator.

Brownies without baking

Servings: 2

Level of difficulty: easy

Ingredients

- 5 dates (dried, without stone)
- 5 Apricots (dried)
- 100 g walnut kernels
- 2 tablespoons cocoa
- ¼ TL Vanilla
- 1 pinch of salt

Preparation

1. Cut the dates and the apricots into small pieces and put them in a blender. Add the walnut kernels, the cocoa, the vanilla, about 2 tablespoons of water and the salt and mix everything well.
2. Form small round balls from the dough. Lay them out on baking paper and put them in the freezer for half an hour.
3. Then you can serve the brownies.

Blueberry cake

Servings: 1 cake

Level of difficulty: easy

Ingredients

- 25 g linseed
- 25 sunflower seeds
- 25 g oat flakes
- 5 dates (pitted)
- 35 ml coconut oil
- 1 banana
- 175 g blueberries
- 80 g cashew nuts

Preparation

1. Peel and slice the banana. Sort and wash the blueberries. Remove small remaining stems.
2. Cut the dates into small pieces and put them in a blender. Add the linseed, sunflower seeds and oat flakes and mix everything together.
3. Melt 1 tablespoon of coconut oil and put it in the blender. Add 2 tablespoons of water. Mix everything again. Add water if necessary.
4. Put the dough into a springform pan.
5. Mix the banana pieces with the blueberries, the cashew nuts and 20 ml coconut oil and put them on the dough.
6. Place the cake in the freezer for 3 hours and then serve.

Cherry pudding with caramel

Servings: 2

Level of difficulty: easy

Ingredients

- 165 g butter
- 140 g sugar
- 225 g cherries
- 50 g flour
- 50 g almonds (ground)
- 1 teaspoon baking powder

Preparation

1. Wash and stone the cherries. Set some cherries aside for decoration.
2. Preheat the oven to 200 degrees (circulating air).
3. Melt 75 g butter. Add 50 g sugar and let everything simmer until the mixture has a golden yellow color.
4. Grease small fireproof molds with butter and place the cherries in the molds.
5. Pour the butter-sugar mixture onto the cherries.
6. Mix the remaining butter with the remaining sugar using a hand mixer. Add flour, almonds and baking powder. Fill the resulting dough into the forms.
7. Place the baking tins in the oven for half an hour.
8. Allow the dough to cool briefly, then loosen carefully with a knife and serve. Garnish the puddings with the cherries put aside.

Muesli Muffins

Servings: 6 Muffins
Level of difficulty: easy

Ingredients

- 100 g spelt flour
- 30 g crunchy muesli
- 125 g mixed berries (fresh or sweet)
- 1 teaspoon baking powder
- 1 egg
- 1 package vanilla sugar
- 2 tablespoons maple syrup
- 100 g yoghurt
- 50 ml oil

Preparation

1. Preheat the oven to 200 degrees (circulating air).
2. Grease a muffin tin with butter or margarine.
3. Select and wash the berries. Use frozen food, defrost them.
4. Mix the flour with the baking powder and the crunchy muesli. Add the egg, vanilla sugar, maple syrup, oil and yogurt. Mix everything well.
5. Fold in the berries.
6. Grease a muffin tin with butter or margarine.
7. Now fill the dough into the molds and put them in the oven for half an hour.
8. Let the muffins cool down a little, then remove them and serve.

Yoghurt and Tangerine Cake

Servings: 1 cake

Level of difficulty: easy

Ingredients

- 5 eggs
- 150 g sugar
- 150 g flour
- 1 knife point of baking powder
- 1 teaspoon lemon peel
- 9 leaves gelatin
- 600 g yoghurt (fat content 1.5%)
- 1 package vanilla sugar
- 250 g mandarins (1 small tin)
- 600 g cream
- 100 g powdered sugar

Preparation

1. Preheat the oven to 170 degrees (circulating air).
2. Mix eggs and sugar with a whisk. Stir in flour, baking powder and lemon peel.
3. Grease a baking tray. Spread the dough on it and bake for 10 minutes.
4. Soak the gelatin in water. Add 2 tablespoons of yoghurt and warm up the mixture slightly on the stove.
5. Mix the remaining yoghurt with the powdered sugar and vanilla sugar. Stir 3 tablespoons of the mixture into the gelatin. Chill the rest.
6. Drain the mandarins. Whip the cream until stiff.
7. As soon as the yoghurt mass becomes firm, stir in the cream and pour the mass onto the cake. Place the mandarins on top.

Quince tart with sprinkles

Servings: 1 Tarte

Level of difficulty: easy

Ingredients

- 1 kg quinces
- 100 g brown cane sugar
- 190 g flour
- 110 g butter
- 1 teaspoon salt
- 1 tablespoon of granulated sugar

Preparation

1. Wash, stone and quarter the quinces.
2. Preheat the oven to 180 degrees (circulating air).
3. Mix the cane sugar with the flour and salt. Warm the butter slightly and work it into the flour mixture. Cover the crumble dough and let it rest.
4. Put the quinces in a pot. Add the granulated sugar and some water and let everything simmer for a few minutes. Remove the liquid with a sieve.
5. Line a tart tin with baking paper. Put the crumbled dough on top and layer the quinces on top.
6. Put the tart in the oven for 45 minutes, then let it cool down and serve. Serve with freshly whipped cream or homemade vanilla sauce.

Cranberry Muffins

Servings: 6 Muffins

Level of difficulty: easy

Ingredients

- 100 g cranberries
- 65 g butter
- 50 g wheat flour
- 125 g flour
- 1 ½ TL Baking powder
- 1 teaspoon bicarbonate of soda
- 115 g sugar
- 1 pinch of salt
- 225 g pumpkin
- 1 egg

Preparation

1. Preheat the oven to 200 degrees (circulating air).
2. Cook the pumpkin for 3 minutes in the microwave on 600 watts. Then cut the pumpkin open, cut into large pieces and puree. Wash and halve the cranberries.
3. Put the two flours, baking powder, baking soda, sugar and salt in a bowl and mix.
4. Add the cranberries, the pumpkin puree, the butter (melt) and the egg. Mix everything well.
5. Grease a muffin tin with butter or margarine.
6. Fill the dough into the molds and bake for half an hour.

pomegranate tart

Servings: 1 Tarte

Level of difficulty: easy

Ingredients

- 100 g butter
- 200 g flour
- 130 g sugar
- 1 package of vanilla pudding
- ½ l milk
- 60 g almond paste (from the health food shop)
- 250 g pomegranate seeds
- 1 package cake glaze (light)
- 100 g pomegranate syrup (from the Asia store)

Preparation

1. Preheat the oven to 180 degrees (circulating air).
2. Grease a tart tin with butter or margarine.
3. Mix butter, flour, 2 tablespoons of sugar and 3 tablespoons of water and place in the tart. Prick the dough with a fork and bake for 40 minutes.
4. Mix the vanilla pudding with the milk, the almond paste and the remaining sugar and spread it on the pastry base.
5. Sprinkle the pomegranate seeds on the pudding.
6. Mix the cake glaze with the pomegranate syrup, sugar and 150 ml water, bring to the boil, cool slightly and apply to the tart.
7. Allow the glaze to set and then serve the tart.

Lemon cake

Servings: 1 cake

Level of difficulty: easy

Ingredients

- 225 g butter
- 225 g sugar
- 3 organic lemons
- 4 eggs
- 250 g wheat flour
- 1 teaspoon baking powder
- 75 g almonds (ground)
- 100 g granulated sugar

Preparation

1. Wash the lemons with hot water and grate the peel. Then cut the lemons open and squeeze them.
2. Grease a cake tin. Preheat the oven to 200 degrees (circulating air).
3. Mix butter, sugar, lemon peel and the egg
4. Mix the flour with the baking powder, the almonds and 2 tablespoons lemon juice. Fold the mixture into the butter and lemon mixture. Put the dough into the form and bake for 45 minutes.
5. Let the dough cool down a little.
6. Mix the remaining lemon juice with the sugar and pour it on the cake.

Kumquat Thyme Cake

Servings: 1 cake
Level of difficulty: easy

Ingredients

- 150 g kumquats
- 190 g brown sugar
- 175 g butter
- 3 eggs
- 125 g wheat flour
- 100 g wholemeal flour
- 1 teaspoon baking powder
- 1 teaspoon thyme (chopped)
- 75 g powdered sugar

Preparation

1. Wash the kumquats and then heat them in a pan with 15 g sugar and 100 ml water and simmer for 5 minutes. Drain the liquid and put aside.
2. Grease a cake tin. Preheat the oven to 160 degrees (circulating air).
3. Mix sugar, butter, eggs, both flours, baking powder and thyme. Add the kumquats to the dough, also 2 tablespoons of the previously poured juice.
4. Pour the mixture into the mold and bake the cake for 60 minutes. Then remove from the oven, let it cool down and serve.

Elderberry pancakes

Servings: 2

Level of difficulty: easy

Ingredients

- 12 bloomed elderberry umbels (alternatively 3 apples)
- 2 eggs
- 100 g flour
- 140 ml milk
- 2 teaspoons sugar
- ½ Organic lemon
- 1 pinch of salt
- some powdered sugar

Preparation

1. Rinse the lemon with hot water and then grate the peel.
2. Wash the elderberry umbels and pat dry with kitchen paper.
3. Separate the eggs. Mix the flour with the milk and the egg yolk. Add lemon zest, sugar and salt.
4. Beat the egg whites until stiff and fold into the dough mixture.
5. Add the flowers to the dough. Pour the dough with a ladle into a pan with hot clarified butter. Bake the pancakes until golden yellow. Turn with a spatula.

Disclaimer

The implementation of all information, instructions and strategies contained in this (e-)book is at your own risk. The author cannot accept liability for any damages of any kind for any legal reason. Liability claims against the author for material or immaterial damages caused by the use or non-use of the information or by the use of incorrect and/or incomplete information are excluded in principle. Therefore, any legal and damage claims are also excluded. This work was compiled and written down with the greatest care and to the best of our knowledge. However, the author accepts no responsibility for the topicality, completeness and quality of the information. Printing errors and misinformation cannot be completely excluded. No legal responsibility or liability of any kind can be assumed for incorrect information provided by the author.

Copyright

Imprint

© MK

2021

1st edition

All rights reserved

Reprinting, even in extracts, is not permitted.

No part of this work may be reproduced, duplicated or distributed in any form without written permission of the author.

Contact us: Matthias Kronawitter, Schnieglinger Str. 94, 90419 Nuremberg, Germany

Made in the USA
Las Vegas, NV
10 June 2021

24517890R10125